Hypothyroidism:
The Unsuspected Illness

Hypothyroidism:
The Unsuspected Illness

By Broda O. Barnes, M.D.,
and Lawrence Galton

1817

HARPER & ROW, PUBLISHERS, New York
Grand Rapids, Philadelphia, St. Louis, San Francisco
London, Singapore, Sydney, Tokyo, Toronto

Manufactured in the United States of America

Library of Congress Cataloging in Publication Data

Barnes, Broda Otto.
    Hypothyroidism: the unsuspected illness.

    Bibliography: p.
    Includes index.
    1. Hypothyroidism.   I.   Galton, Lawrence,
joint author.   II.   Title. [DNLM: 1.   Hypo-
thyroidism--Popular works.   WK265 B261h]
RC657.B34   616.4'44   75-29251
ISBN 0-690-01029-X

    04 05 06 HAD 50 49 48 47 46 45

Contents

A Personal Message
to the Reader

FORTY PERCENT of the American people—four of every ten children and adults—today are suffering needlessly and many are dying for lack of an ingredient vital for health.

Is the ingredient unknown? No. Or unavailable? No.

For years, medicine has recognized the role of the deficiency in some areas of health and disease and has had clues to its great importance in many other areas.

But the knowledge too often has not been used—and still is not being used—because of the unreliablity of laboratory tests that have failed to show the deficiency even when doctors could see its manifestations clearly enough in patients before them. And while laboratory tests have erred and have misled both doctors and patients, patients have suffered.

After spending thirty-five years of a medical career

with the problem and with thousands of patients who have had it—and with learning from my own and from the studies of others how the problem can be recognized readily and then treated easily, effectively, and inexpensively—my purpose in writing this book is to alert you and as many others as I can reach so that a powerful but largely unused weapon for many of our ills will no longer be overlooked.

—Broda O. Barnes, M.D., Ph.D.

Dr. Barnes passed away on November 1, 1988, at age 82. His work transformed the lives of many of his patients. People who had suffered for years and spent large sums of money on treatment were finally able to find relief with the simple, effective methods advocated by Dr. Barnes. With his second wife Helen, he established the Broda O. Barnes, M.D. Research Foundation to continue his research. It exists today as a resource for the general public as well as medical professionals. To obtain additional information, please contact the foundation at the address below.

Broda O. Barnes, M.D.
Research Foundation, Inc.
P.O. Box 98
Trumbull, CT 06611
(203) 261-2101

Hypothyroidism:
The Unsuspected Illness

I

The Many Faces of Thyroid Deficiency

- A young housewife who feels rundown, tires easily, is sleepy much of the time, and strangely oversensitive to cold weather.
- A middle-aged man who has managed to distinguish himself in his career by fighting all his life against his low energy reserve but now has become tired of fighting and convinced there must be some physical explanation for his problem even though none has ever been found and more than once he has been told to consult a psychiatrist and more than once has done so without benefit.
- A victim of severe recurrent headaches.
- A barren couple.
- A child or adult unusually prone to infections, particulary respiratory, but not limited to them.

- A sufferer from severe rheumatic pain and a potential heart attack victim.

- A woman whose skin is abnormally rough, scaly, almost fishlike and patients with other skin problems, including eczema, psoriasis, and acne.

- At least one man or woman in a state of severe mental depression.

- A woman with a menstrual problem—painful flow, or irregular flow, or sometimes excessive flow that suggests possible need for hysterectomy.

These are a few of the people who will pass through my waiting room on almost any routine day. There is one striking common fact about them: Varied as are their symptoms, the cause of their illness in every case is the same—low thyroid function.

Of all the sly, subtle problems that can affect physical or mental health, none is more common than thyroid gland disturbance. And none is more readily—and inexpensively—corrected. Yet none is more often untreated and even unsuspected

In my years of experience, I have seen patients who for much or all of their lives have had health difficulties that should have suggested the possibility of low thyroid function (hypothyroidism) and whose whole lives could have been changed by simple treatment for it. Yet the thyroid disturbance went unsuspected in many and in others, even when briefly suspected, went unverified and untreated. Nor is it difficult to appreciate why this could —and still does—happen so often.

Sources of Neglect and Confusion

It's impossible to overemphasize the importance of the thyroid, a small, butterfly-shaped gland located in the neck and weighing less than an ounce. It is the thyroid which controls metabolism—the process by which food is transformed into energy and many vital chemical changes take place. Minute thyroid secretions, something less than a spoonful a year, are responsible for much of the body's heat production. They help maintain the circulatory system and blood volume. They are necessary for muscle health. They heighten sensitivity of nerves. Every organ, every tissue, every cell is affected by the hormone secretions of the gland.

That severe hypothyroidism can have devastating effects has long been appreciated. A cretin child, born with a grossly defective thyroid gland, will remain a dwarf and become an idiot unless given thyroid to make up for the gland's total or near-total failure to produce secretions.

A severely hypothyroid adult, whose gland produces grossly inadequate amounts of secretions, may have a "moon-shaped" face, coarse features, thick nostrils and lips, slow and thick speech, and suffer from weakness and listlessness to the point of apathy.

Fortunately, extreme hypothyroidism is rare. But mild or moderate hypothyroidism is far from rare. And the results of it can be confusing. There are none of the classic gross changes in physical features that occur with the extreme form. Instead, there can be varied symptoms that may seem, on the surface, far removed from the thyroid.

One of the most common symptoms is fatigue. It can

vary from relatively mild to severe. It may come on so slowly that a victim, feeling no sudden, precipitous decline in energy level, may come to accept fatigability as—for him—a virtually normal state.

In one case, low thyroid function may give rise to fatigue alone; in another, fatigue may be present but of lesser importance compared with, say, recurrent severe headaches. In other cases, there may be other symptoms, sometimes a whole complex of symptoms. Repeated infections, skin problems, menstrual disturbances of many kinds, memory disturbances, concentration difficulties, depression, paranoid symptoms—these are just a few of many possible manifestations.

Unless it is recognized that low thyroid function can have many effects which may vary considerably from one victim to another, the possibility that this is where the trouble may lie may never even be considered. In my experience, many patients with problems labeled "psychosomatic"—and many who have been classified as being hypochondriacs—are victims of unrecognized hypothyroidism.

Failing Tests

Another source of confusion has been the failure of standard thyroid function tests to detect hypothyroidism reliably. The basal metabolism test, for example, one of the very first to be used, checks thyroid function by measuring oxygen consumed when the body is at rest —doing nothing but sustaining itself. When hypothyroidism is pronounced, the test may pick it up but otherwise may not. There are, as we shall see, good reasons why it is—virtually has to be—often inaccurate.

Other tests, such as protein-bound iodine and radio-active iodine uptake, may also not always be dependable, although for a long time they were considered reliable. In fact, *The Medical Letter,* an independent medical-evaluation bulletin for physicians, recently has warned that many commonly used drugs—and even shampoo and skin antiseptic compounds—can upset test results.

A Simple Home Test

Some years ago, seeking a better index of thyroid function, I began to use and still use a simple temperature test. It costs nothing. It requires only an ordinary thermometer. Any patient can self-administer the test at home in ten minutes—and, in fact, the test is best carried out at home. The test must be done in a certain way but it is a very simple procedure. Details about the test have been published in the medical literature. Not all doctors by any means are using it yet, but more and more are. (Later in this book, you will find specific instructions for carrying out the test if you wish to do so, along with a full explanation of the basis for the test.)

It is a test for basal—or, at-rest—temperature which differs from the everyday oral and rectal temperature reading in that the entire body must be completely at rest. There is a definite range for normal basal temperature. Below that range, low thyroid function is indicated.

The temperature test has checked out against the basal metabolism and other thyroid tests and has revealed hypothyroidism when the other tests have done so *and* when they have *failed* to do so. And when patients with low basal temperature have had thyroid treatment, their symptoms have disappeared as their basal temperature has climbed.

In thousands of patients, use of the basal temperature test to detect hypothyroidism and then to correct it—starting with very small doses of thyroid medication and increasing them, if necessary, until retesting has shown the temperature rising—has led to gratifying results.

Some Patients Who Have Responded

One patient who illustrates well how so many manifestations of low thyroid function may sometimes appear in the same individual and go undiagnosed is a thirty-seven-year-old woman I saw six years ago. Her primary complaint then was extreme fatigue. She was having great difficulty caring for her three children, aged seven to twelve. She was also markedly depressed.

Actually, a first possible indication of thyroid deficiency had come when she was in the third grade and had to be sent home repeatedly from school with severe headaches. Another came when she started her menses at age eleven, flowed heavily, experienced severe cramps, and lost several days each month from school. Still another was her tendency to develop far more than the usual number of colds and upper respiratory infections. As a freshman in high school, she developed severe pneumonia complicated by empyema, a collection of pus between lung and rib cage. She had to be hospitalized for two months, was out of school for a year, and an ugly scar at the bottom of the ribs on her back offers testimony to prolonged drainage.

In college, an astute physician realized that she needed thyroid and her health improved on thyroid therapy, but soon another physician discontinued the medication seeing no paticular need for it. Her obstetrician put her back on thyroid during her first pregnancy, but later another physician stopped the medication.

I examined her thoroughly, did blood and other laboratory tests to exclude other possible factors, and had her take her basal temperature at home. I could hardly be surprised when it proved to be below normal.

Her response to thyroid therapy didn't come overnight, of course. But over a period of several weeks, she began to notice that she no longer felt fatigued immediately after arising in the morning and over the next several weeks she felt a progressive increase in vigor. Her depression began to lift, too. Over a period of several months, her menses became regular. The next winter she experienced only one cold instead of the usual repeated wintertime respiratory problems, and the winter after that she was free of any respiratory infection. On continued thyroid therapy, just enough to maintain her basal temperature in the normal range, she is today a thoroughly healthy and effective wife and mother.

A man in his midforties had fought the handicap of excessive fatigue all of his life—and well enough to have become professor and chairman of his department at a major university. For years he had needed a minimum of ten hours' sleep a night plus frequent rest periods during the day. He was slow in his actions and slow in conversation. His slowness—since he was a brilliant man—had been regarded by his colleagues as an indication only of a deliberate, meticulous personality.

He sought help when, during an administrative crisis at the university, he felt that he was on the verge of total exhaustion. Like many hypothyroid patients I have seen, he told me that he felt as if he had been "born tired." And he added: "I am just tired now of being tired and of having to fight so hard against it."

The basal temperature test did not leave the slightest doubt about his low thyroid function. He responded, as expected, to thyroid therapy. Within a few months, he was delighted not only with his increased vigor but also with finding that his thought processes were faster, he was getting more fun and excitement out of his work, and, needing less sleep, he had time for avocational activities.

More Patients

I have seen many "hopelessly lazy" children who weren't basically lazy at all and who, when their thyroid deficiency was detected and adequately treated, lost their laziness.

Headaches can have many causes. But repeatedly I have seen hypothyroid patients with headaches associated with easy fatigability; their headaches have been reduced greatly in frequency and severity and in some cases eliminated entirely once their hypothyroidism was corrected.

Many skin disorders in hypothyroid patients have yielded to thyroid therapy. One baby comes vividly to mind even after more than twenty years. He was seven months of age when I first saw him. He had bleeding eczema covering virtually his whole body. Since birth he had been kept in a straitjacket to keep him from scratching himself to death by hemorrhage. Two hospitalizations and repeated dermatological consultations had been to no avail. Five months of thyroid therapy cleared his skin.

Psoriasis is a serious, often disfiguring skin problem that still remains mysterious. Not all but at least some patients with the disease have responded to thyroid treatment. One, a retired dean of the University of Denver, had had psoriasis for fifty years; it cleared entirely on thyroid therapy.

I have seen many patients with acne—teen-agers and adults—who, when they also had hypothyroidism, experienced marked improvement and even complete clearing of the skin on thyroid treatment. And results in those with chronic boils have often been remarkable as thyroid treatment has built resistance to bacteria ever-present on the skin.

Chronic or recurrent infection of one kind or another has been "the story of my life" for many patients with thyroid deficiency. One man, seventy-nine years old when first seen, had had a left ear draining pus since childhood. For twenty years, he had suffered from a bone infection which oozed pus continuously from his left thigh. Three months after he was started on thyroid treatment, his leg infection cleared; after a year, his ear was clear.

I have seen many children who suffered from repeated colds followed by complications such as tonsillitis, sinusitis, ear and mastoid infections, who needed repeated antibiotic treatment and went right on getting new infections until their hypothyroidism was treated.

Menstrual disorders may stem from fibroids, ovarian cysts, cervical polyps and other organic causes, but in most cases no such physical abnormalities are found. But many women with menstrual problems have proved to be hypothyroid and among them, my records show, about 90 percent have experienced relief of painful menstruation following thyroid therapy, and cure rates have been equally high for those with irregular cycles and others with excessive bleeding.

But Is It Psychogenic?
Must It be Mental Deterioration?

On a warm day a few years ago, a middle-aged housewife was brought into my office by her husband, a professional man who had happened to read some of my reports on low thyroid function in the medical literature. He felt that before carrying her off to a mental institution for extended treatment—a recommendation of both family physician and psychiatrist after fruitless attempts to help her—it would do no harm to have her thyroid function investigated.

In addition to the pajamas and heavy bathrobe she wore, she was wrapped in a heavy blanket, yet she sat before me shaking with cold. For a year, she had experienced loss of appetite, loss of weight, sleeplessness, eye inflammation, hoarseness, nervousness, poor memory, difficulty in thinking. Even before that, she had become frightened of crowds and wouldn't leave the house. She was unable to cook because she could not remember what ingredients she had already added.

There had been extensive examinations and laboratory tests. All results were within the normal range. Seemingly, hers must be a mental problem. Yet, what had been overlooked by her previous physicians was that mental conditions are common in thyroid disorders; indeed, British studies had demonstrated this even before the turn of the century. Her shivering and shaking on a warm day, despite being well wrapped, was in itself a clue to hypothyroidism.

When her low thyroid function was confirmed by temperature test, she was started on thyroid therapy with the advice that it would be at the very least a month before any improvement could be anticipated. Meanwhile, to make the family feel better, she was referred to a competent neurologist to rule out the possibility of any serious neurological problem. The neurologist found nothing and advised her to continue with thyroid therapy. Improvement did begin in a month and continued. Within several months, she was free of all symptoms, including her fears.

An example of what might erroneously be supposed to be mental deterioration associated with aging is the case of a sixty-five-year-old woman whose history suggested that she might have had some relatively mild manifestations, particularly a tendency to undue fatigue, of hypothyroidism for much of her life. But there had been serious difficulties only for the past three years. For each of the past three winters, she had required hospitalization and had been given shock treatment for depression accompanied by mental aberrations. She was better each summer, but slumped again each winter. This suggested the possibility of thyroid deficiency since more thyroid is needed in cold weather to step up the body's burning of fuel required to combat cold. Her hypothyroidism was confirmed by temperature test and she was started on thyroid therapy. She has now passed through four winters without difficulty, full of gratitude for her escape from further shock therapy.

I have seen many other problems, otherwise mysterious and unyielding, associated with low thyroid function and responsive to thyroid treatment to restore thyroid levels to normal. And it is gratifying to report that so have other physicians, when they are suspicious of the possibility that hypothyroidism may be at fault.

Recently, for example, Mayo Clinic physicians have found that poor equilibrium, muscle aches and weakness, some hearing disturbances, and nervous system changes leading to burning and prickling sensations are due in some cases to reduced thyroid activity and respond to thyroid therapy. Recently, too, in University of North Carolina School of Medicine studies, hypothyroidism has been found associated with varied mental disturbances, including depression, memory loss, and difficulties in concentrating.

Thyroid and the Heart

Coming as I did into medicine with special training in the functioning of the thyroid gland—prior to medical school I took my Ph.D. in physiology, did research on the thyroid for my doctoral dissertation, and taught endocrinology at the University of Chicago—I was prepared to find faulty thyroid functioning capable of producing a wide array of problems.

But I was not prepared particularly for the finding that hypothyroidism could play any significant role in heart problems and that thyroid therapy could offer any protection against "coronaries."

In 1950, however, a friend had a heart attack. He lived at a distance, had not been a patient of mine, but after his attack, when I visited him and went over his history, I found that for some years he had suffered symptoms of hypothyroidism for which he had not sought medical advice.

Suddenly, then, it struck me that in my medical practice, which had attracted a sizeable proportion of patients with thyroid problems who had been treated with thyroid, heart attacks had been conspicuously absent—at a time when they were rising rapidly in the general population.

Was this coincidence? Cholesterol was supposed to be a culprit, a major culprit according to some investigators. The thyroid had much to do with controlling blood cholesterol levels. It seemed to me that the possible role of thyroid deficiency in heart disease needed to be investigated.

Beginning in 1950 each new adult patient, in addition to testing for thyroid function, was questioned about any history of heart disease in the family and received a chest X-ray for heart size, an electrocardiogram and other heart studies. There was no reduction of fats or cholesterol-rich foods in the diet. The only change in daily routine was the taking of thryoid medication for hypothyroidism.

When I had accumulated a sizeable number of patients followed over an extended period of years, I made an analysis. There were 490 women aged thirty to fifty-nine. Based on national statistics, in this many women over the period of time, eight cases of heart disease were to be expected. None had developed.

There were 172 high-risk women—that is, women with high blood pressure or high cholesterol levels or both; in that group of women, based on national statistics, at least seven cases of heart disease were to be expected. None had developed.

There were 182 women aged sixty and over and in that group eight cases were to be expected. None had developed.

There were 382 men, aged thirty to fifty-nine, and, based on national statistics, it was to be expected that at least twelve would develop heart disease. Only one did.

There were 186 high-risk men; nineteen cases of heart disease were to be expected; there were only two.

There were 157 men, aged sixty and over; eighteen cases were to be expected; only one developed.

Thus, with seventy-two cases of heart disease to be expected based on national statistics and with only four actually developing, treatment for hypothyroidism produced 94 percent protection.

The New Population

I am convinced that we are seeing today many more people with low thyroid function than ever before, and that the rising incidence of heart attacks is related to the rising incidence of hypothyroidism. There are some indications, too, very much worth exploring, that our rising incidence of lung cancer and of the serious lung disease emphysema may be associated with the increase in hypothyroidism which now may be affecting as many as 40 percent of the population and in another decade may affect half the population. For we have today a new population—and it accounts for the rising incidence of thyroid deficiency.

While attention has been focused on the many changes in the environment brought about by modern technology, perhaps the greatest change of all has been in man himself.

Up to this century, more than half of all children died before reaching adulthood. Adults were largely those who were resistant to infectious diseases. Survival depended upon resistance; medicine had little to offer. It was not unusual that Beethoven, for example, was one of only three survivors out of seven births.

Now adults are composed of two groups—those resistant to infection and those who, although susceptible, have escaped death as the result of modern medicine. This second group is the "new" population. Its members not only have a proclivity toward infectious disease due in no small part to a hereditary proneness to thyroid deficiency which lowers resistance to infections but, as a result, they also have a proneness to heart disease and, it would seem, to other degenerative diseases such as emphysema and lung cancer.

Heart attacks, indeed, were first associated with infectious disease during World War II, when there were 866 such attacks in American servicemen below the age of forty. Only two important correlations were found: a family history of the disease and a history of previous pneumonia in the men themselves. Pneumonia is an indication of low resistance to infectious diseases, in most cases as a result of thyroid deficiency.

There is much more evidence to substantiate the fact that we have a new population and to support the association of hypothyroidism with heart and other degenerative diseases.

What you will be reading in the following pages will seem like, and in fact has been, a medical detective story. I am certainly not the only detective involved. I have followed many of the clues but many other researchers have done so concurrently and independently of me —and some long before, although their work until recently has been largely overlooked.

It must no longer be overlooked.

It has too much of value to offer.

To fight malaise, general ill health, and outright disease with drugs that are nonbiological weapons, not natural to the body, is fine when we have nothing else. Aspirin may relieve a headache, antibiotics an infection, nitroglycerin the chest pain cry of the heart, but we don't get headaches, infections, or heart disease from *lack* of aspirin, antibiotics, or nitroglycerin in our systems.

If we get them—and much else—because of the reduced secretions of a low-functioning thyroid gland, we are far more likely to combat them effectively and safely by giving the body what is lacking: its own potent biological weapon.

2

The Vital—
and Errant—Gland

UNTIL ABOUT a century ago, the single controlling force for all of the complex processes that go on in the human body was thought to be the nervous system. But there were too many phenomena that, when carefully analyzed, seemed to have no relationship to the nervous system, too many differences in people—in size and energy, for example—that could not be accounted for satisfactorily in terms of nervous activity alone.

The explanation was to be found in certain glands, the endocrines, of which the thyroid is one and, in fact, one of the first to be discovered.

There is an old medical saying that just a few grams of thyroid hormone can make the difference between an idiot and an Einstein. It aptly characterizes the thyroid's role as a quickener of the tempo of life.

All of the endocrine glands play remarkable roles in

the body economy. Unlike the many millions of other glands such as the sweat glands in the skin, the salivary glands in the mouth, the tear glands in the eyes, which perform only local functions, the endocrines pour their hormone secretions into the bloodstream which carries them to all parts of the body.

From the pea-size pituitary gland at the base of the brain come hormones that influence growth, sexual development, uterine contraction in childbirth, and milk release afterward. The adrenals, rising like mushrooms from atop the kidneys, pour out more than a score of hormones, including hydrocortisone and adrenaline needed for the body's response to stress and injury.

Also in the endocrine system are the sex glands —ovaries and testes; the pineal gland in the brain whose hormones are thought to play a role in nerve and brain functioning; the thymus behind the breastbone which appears to be involved in establishing the body's immunity system; and areas in the pancreas, the islets of Langerhans, which secrete insulin.

The Thyroid

It is the thyroid gland, lying in front of the throat below the Adam's apple and just above the breastbone, which regulates the rate at which the body utilizes oxygen and controls the rate at which various organs function and the speed with which the body utilizes food.

In a way, the thyroid, through its hormone secretions, functions as a kind of thermostat. Each individual cell in the body is much like a microscopic power plant: it burns food and sets energy free, some of the energy being released as heat. Thyroid secretion is essential for the operation of the cell and, in effect, determines how hot the fire gets in the cell and the speed of activity in the cell. The term "metabolism" refers to the fires within body cells.

The influence of thyroid secretion on body processes and other organs is almost incredibly widespread and important. When the thyroid gland is removed from an otherwise normal animal, all metabolic activity is reduced. A decrease in heat production begins—in rabbits, for example, within five to seven days after the operation. By about the third week, metabolism reaches its lowest level, 35 to 40 percent below normal, a reduction corresponding to that seen in severe cases of hypothyroidism in humans. The metabolic rate may be restored to normal or even to above normal by the administration of thyroid substance.

After removal of the thyroid gland, excess amounts of water, salts, and protein are retained within the body. Blood cholesterol also goes up.

The thyroid plays an important role in growth processes. Tadpoles, deprived of thyroid, fail to metamorphose into frogs, but they do so at an accelerated rate when excess thyroid is administered. If a just-hatched tadpole is given extra thyroid hormone, it turns prematurely into an adult frog about the size of a fly.

In the human, growth and maturation fail to take place normally when the thyroid is absent or functioning far below normal. Children lacking normal thyroid function may remain small; their stature can be improved considerably by thyroid medication started at an early age. Growth of the skin, hair, and nails may be retarded in thyroid deficiency and accelerated again by thyroid treatment. Healing of bone is delayed in thyroid deficiency. A rather severe anemia may develop in severe hypothyroidism. Thyroid hormone is essential for normal nervous system functioning and reaction time, and hypothyroidism may produce slow reactions and mental sluggishness. Muscle health too is dependent on thyroid secretion and with marked thyroid deficiency the muscles may become sluggish and infiltrated with fat.

There are interrelationships between the thyroid and the other endocrine glands. When, for example, thyroid deficiency is marked, the effect on the sex glands is shown by subnormal sexual development and function and impairment of libido. In hypothyroid women, menstrual disturbances are present frequently.

The Extremes

Fortunately, cretinism and myxedema, the extreme forms of hypothyroidism, are relatively rare. We have mentioned them earlier but they deserve a little more detailed look because they so clearly indicate the importance of proper thyroid function.

Cretinism is a condition found in infants and children resulting from a deficiency of thyroid hormone during fetal or early life. The thyroid gland may be entirely absent or greatly reduced in size.

In a cretin child, the skin is thick, dry, wrinkled, and sallow; the tongue is enlarged; the lips thickened; the mouth open and drooling; the face broad; the nose flat;

the feet and hands puffy. The child is dull and apathetic. Although a cretin child may be unusually large at birth, development is defective and, if the child is untreated, he becomes small for his age in childhood and a dwarf in adulthood, suffering mental retardation along with growth failure. With early and adequate thyroid hormone treatment for cretinism, growth may become normal and mental status may improve.

Myxedema is the reaction in adulthood to lack of thyroid hormone, either because the thyroid gland wastes away or has to be removed, or because of failure of the pituitary gland to stimulate thyroid activity.

Myxedema brings with it gradual personality changes along with marked physical changes. They include a general, progressive slowing of mental and physical activity, an increase in weight, a decrease in appetite. Facial changes occur and may progress steadily to produce a masklike appearance, as the skin becomes thick and somewhat rigid, interfering with expression.

The skin also becomes dry, cold, rough, and scaly; it appears waterlogged and swollen. Characteristically, the upper eyelids become waterlogged or edematous and the eyebrows may be elevated because of efforts to keep the eyes open.

The hair becomes coarse, brittle, and tends to fall out; the nails become brittle and grow slowly; there is sensitivity to cold with feelings of being chilly in rooms of normal temperature; and perspiration is decreased or absent even during hot weather. Many myxedematous patients are troubled by joint pains and stiffness. Resistance to infection is decreased, wounds heal slowly, and ulcers may be persistent.

The tongue and lips become large and thick and, because of this and also because of retarded mental reaction and decreased muscular coordination, the speech becomes slow, thick, and clumsy and may resemble that of a slightly intoxicated person.

A myxedema victim generally appears slow, drowsy, and placid. Normal mental effort cannot be maintained. A tendency to drop off to sleep during the day may be present. Anemia is usually present in some form; constipation is nearly always present; depression is common as is decline in libido and sexual function.

Yet, all of these manifestations are dramatically controllable when thyroid is administered in suitable dosage.

Milder Forms

As cretinism and myxedema demonstrate, virtually no system of the body may escape the effects of severe lack or complete absence of thyroid hormone secretions. Yet even in extreme forms of hypothyroidism, there are variations in manifestations, some being more overt and troublesome than others.

Hypothyroidism of milder degree can be far more subtle. It, too, may affect many systems of the body but not all to the same degree. One patient may have manifestations that another does not. It is as if there are variations among individuals in organs and systems which are most susceptible to thyroid deficiency. Such varying susceptibility is, of course, well known in allergy. In the allergic, a food, pollen, or other material to which there is sensitivity may produce varying symptoms depending upon the "target" organs affected, the organs with greater allergic susceptibility. If, for example, the nose is a target organ, there may be nasal congestion, watery discharge, and sneezing, as in hay fever; if the skin is the target, there may be rash, hives, or eczema; if the bronchial tubes are the target, there is the wheezing of bronchial asthma.

The relative frequency of symptoms and signs of hypothyroidism has been studied by two medical investigators in two different series of patients and is shown in the following list:

Incidence of Symptoms and Signs of Hypothyroidism*

	Study A % of 77 cases	Study B % of 100 cases
Weakness	99	98
Dry skin	97	79
Coarse skin	97	70
Lethargy	91	85
Slow speech	91	56
Edema (swelling) of eyelids	90	86
Sensation of cold	89	95
Decreased sweating	89	68
Cold skin	83	80
Thick tongue	82	60
Edema of face	79	95
Coarseness of hair	76	75
Heart enlargement	68	—**
Pallor of skin	67	50
Impaired memory	66	65
Constipation	61	54

Gain in weight	59	76
Loss of hair	57	41
Pallor of lips	57	50
Labored or difficult breathing	55	72
Swelling of feet	55	57
Hoarseness	52	74
Loss of appetite	45	40
Nervousness	35	51
Excessive menstruation	32	33
Deafness	30	40
Palpitations	31	23
Poor heart sounds	30	—
Pain over the heart	25	16
Poor vision	24	—
Changes in back of eye	20	—
Painful menstruation	18	—
Loss of weight	13	9
Emotional instability	11	—
Choking sensation	9	—
Fineness of hair	9	—
Cyanosis (bluish discoloration of skin)	9	—
Difficulty in swallowing	3	—
Brittle nails	—	41
Depression	—	60
Muscle weakness	—	61
Muscle pain	—	36
Joint pain	—	29
Burning or tingling sensations	—	56
Heat intolerance	—	2
Slowing of mental activity	—	49
Slow movements	—	73

*From J. H. Means, L. J. DeGroot, and J. B. Stanbury, *The Thyroid and Its Diseases*, McGraw-Hill, 1963, pgs. 321-22.

**Dash means not reported found.*

The list shows not only great variation in incidence of various symptoms and signs but also that hypothyroidism is capable of producing some seemingly paradoxical effects. For example, it may lead to coarseness of the hair in some cases, fineness of hair in others; to cold sensations in most cases but to heat intolerance in a few; to gain in weight in some cases and to loss in others.

In a very mild hypothyroid patient, any one, or several, or even many of the symptoms listed may be present and yet may be so subtle that the patient is not particularly aware of them.

From Childhood On

Relatively mild thyroid deficiency in a newborn may not be readily apparent. Such a child may be more quiet than others and may sleep more. Sometimes, the face may be broader than normal and may rarely change expression, breathing may be somewhat noisy, and the baby may appear to have a cold much or all of the time.

Preschool children with low thyroid function may have a somewhat dull and apathetic appearance and be less active than normal youngsters. Yet, paradoxically, a few will be very nervous, hyperactive, and unusually agressive. Emotional problems are frequent. A low thyroid child may cry for no apparent reason and object vigorously to any restrictions. Temper tantrums are common, probably related to undue fatigue. The child may sleep longer than other youngsters of his or her age, be a slow starter in the morning, have a short attention span, and flit from one activity to another. And infections are common.

Once a low-thyroid child starts to school, other problems may arise. With low energy endowment, the child may lack self-confidence and have difficulties in associating successfully with other children. He may be unable to sit quietly and study and his progress in school may be slow. His susceptibility to respiratory infections from other youngsters has increased and with his resistance weakened by low thyroid function he acquires far more than his fair share. Removal of tonsils may end repeated bouts of tonsillitis but does nothing to overcome low resistance to other respiratory infections, sore throats, earaches, and the like.

With puberty other problems may develop. Sports may further deplete low energy endowment; so may any part-time jobs; and school failure may occur. Girls beginning the menstrual cycle may develop low-grade anemia as the result of periodic blood loss, and this further depletes their energy.

Although in childhood growth may be stunted by a marked thyroid deficiency, there may be a seemingly paradoxical effect of a minor deficiency at puberty. The individual may become unusually tall. Growth stops with the closing of the growth centers at the end of each long bone. Thyroid hormone plays a part in causing these centers to close normally. With thyroid deficiency, growth may continue for some time. For many years, I have noted that individuals of either sex who are well over six feet in height consistently run basal temperatures a little below normal range, indicating low thyroid function.

In adulthood, many of the effects of low thyroid function experienced in childhood may be carried over and new ones may emerge.

The "problem" child—who wasn't really a problem in the sense of being deliberately perverse and difficult but rather was experiencing the effects of low thyroid function—may become an adult who all too easily may be mislabeled a "neurotic" or "hypochondriac" because of persistent or even accentuated fatigue, headaches, circulatory disturbances, and other manifestations of low thyroid function.

Why Is Hypothyroidism on the Rise?

The thyroid gland is a factory. To produce its secretions it must, of course, have raw material. If it lacks adequate raw material, its production slumps. When this happens, when the slump is great enough, there may be signals from elsewhere in the body that amount to exhortations for the gland to increase its output. Trying to oblige, the gland may increase in size in a kind of blind effort to add to its output even though it cannot increase production for lack of raw material.

The gland may enlarge until a noticeable lump may appear in the throat. And the swelling, or goiter, may become large enough to interfere with breathing or swallowing.

For a long time, it was mistakenly believed that certain "stale" waters produced goiter. Michelangelo, in the course of painting the Sistine Chapel, wrote: "I have grown a goiter while dwelling in these dens similar to the cat's from the stagnant pools of Lombardy."

It is well known that the real cause of such simple goiter is lack of sufficient iodine in the soil and drinking water. The thyroid gland is the principal user of iodine in the body. In a normal person, dietary iodine is absorbed from the gut into the blood and then, in the thyroid, is removed from the blood, "trapped" in the gland, and incorporated there into compounds which in turn are assembled into thyroid hormone secretions.

The average iodine intake of a normal adult on an ordinary diet in a nongoiter region is about 0.03 milligrams, or 0.0000001 ounce, a day. This tiny amount is only about one-seventh of what is needed for daily thyroid hormone production, but the body practices great economy and re-uses much of its iodine store repeatedly in producing hormone secretions.

In goiter regions, not even the 0.03 milligram per day is available in the food and water. Goiter regions are to be found all over the world. No continent is free of them. Generally they are the mountainous and inland areas of the globe. A high incidence of goiter is found in the Himalayas in Asia, in the regions of the Alps and the Carpathian and Pyrenees mountains in Europe, and in the high plateaus of the Andes in South America. In North America, the goiter zone is the Great Lakes basin and the area of the St. Lawrence River, extending westward through Minnesota, the Dakotas, and the neighboring Canadian territory as far as the northwest and including Oregon, Washington, and British Columbia. This great belt extends an arm southward in the Rocky Mountain area and another in the Appalachian area.

It is in such high and inland areas that, through the ages, the soil has yielded most or all of its soluble iodine content to water on the way to the sea. In areas close to the sea, the soil as well as drinking water is usually rich in iodine. Fruits and vegetables grown in such soil contain iodine in abundance and this is equally true of sea food.

The incidence of goiter in high and inland areas in the past was extremely great. In some Alpine areas, for example, the incidence approached 100 percent. It has never been that high in the United States but it has been high enough to be worrisome. As late as 1936, when the Committee on Goiter of the Wisconsin State Medical Society conducted a survey of the approximate 554,000 school children in Wisconsin, 100,000 showed an abnormal thyroid gland.

The most important discovery in relation to goiter was that the disorder could be prevented by administration of iodine. The iodine could be added to community water supply in goiter regions, or it could be administered in the form of tablets or drops, or it could be taken in the form of iodized salt. Today, use of iodized salt is the most widely accepted method of goiter prevention.

But if goiter now is far less of a problem, not so hypothyroidism. For low thyroid function can be—and commonly is—present in the absence of goiter.

It has long been established that just as goiter is often found among members of the same family, so is low thyroid function without goiter. This familial pattern indicates that there may be a genetically determined biochemical disturbance in the functioning of the gland. Many people, by inheritance, may thus have a special sensitivity to lack of iodine which causes them to develop goiter when iodine intake is inadequate. But even when the iodine intake is adequate, genetic influences may make them prone to have low thyroid function.

One might expect that over a period of time, as low thyroid individuals married others with normal thyroid function, the low thyroid trait would disappear or at least become less common. But experience over many years has shown that more often than not one thyroid-deficient person marries another, helping to perpetuate and even increase the incidence of the trait.

This idea is not as strange as it may seem at first blush, if we consider the fact that unless a courtship is a whirl-wind affair, individuals with similar amounts of energy tend to pair off. It would be difficult for a low thyroid person with a tendency to be more easily fatigued and to require more sleep to date a normal person several nights a week and still function adequately by day; and the normal partner, if attracted at first to the other, would be likely soon to have second thoughts. If, in fact, individuals with marked differences in energy endowment should marry, some would, sooner or later, seek divorce.

I recall one patient, a man who had been grossly over-weight and had had just enough energy to get through a day's work. With thyroid therapy and change of diet, he lost weight, became energetic, and then returned almost a year later complaining that he couldn't go on with his wife. She was tired, cross, unwilling to go out evenings.

When he was reminded that he used to come home from work, eat, read a paper, and go to bed, he realized that the present incompatability had grown out of the change in his energy level, and that perhaps what was needed was some attention to the thyroid status of his wife.

Beyond the tendency of low thyroids to find them-selves attracted to each other and to marry and thus preserve the trait, there is, noted earlier, the tremen-dous increased ability of modern medicine to preserve the low thyroids, to combat their susceptibility to infectious diseases and severe complications that might otherwise be lethal.

How Frequent Is Low Thyroid Function?

Because commonly used tests for thyroid function are not accurate particularly when it comes to mild and even some moderate forms of hypothyroidism and many if not most of those with low thyroid function remain undiscovered, there are no accurate figures on the incidence.

Dr. Paul Starr of the University of California, one of the country's early and most prominent investigators of thyroid function, used to say about fifty years ago that he believed, on the basis of his experience and use of then-available thyroid function tests, that about 10 percent of the population was hypothyroid.

I recall well that when I organized a student health service at the University of Denver in 1941, I found indications of low thyroid function in about 20 percent of the students.

The introduction of antibiotics about 1945 saved millions of hypothyroid children from premature death, allowing them later to reproduce and pass on to their children a low thyroid function tendency, and this accounts for a marked recent increase in hypothyroidism.

I am convinced, as I indicated earlier, that as many as 40 percent of Americans today are affected by some degree of hypothyroidism. They include many of those with a wide variety of complaints such as undue fatigue, chronic headaches, menstrual difficulties, skin problems, repeated infections, and other problems we shall be looking into in detail in the chapters that follow. They include many being fed stimulants, tranquilizers, or other medications which serve only to somewhat dampen symptoms without getting at the cause. They include many who are considered neurotics or hypochondriacs. They include many who are being victimized by heart disease and perhaps other major degenerative diseases.

Hypothyroidism, though widely prevalent, too often is going unrecognized. And we shall see why—and what you can do to determine whether it may be a problem for you or for someone in your family—in the next chapter.

3

The Flaw in Diagnosis . . . and Overcoming It

IT MAY SEEM almost incredible that scientists can sit quietly on earth and follow the activity of the heart of a man walking on the moon and yet they have had so much difficulty in measuring the amount of thyroid hormone necessary for health and in developing effective and reliable tests to determine when thyroid function is inadequate.

The lack of any such test has troubled many physicians. It troubled me almost from the moment I became a physician because of the particular type of training I had received before entering medicine.

In 1930, I arrived as an enthusiastic, ambitious graduate student at the physiology department of the University of Chicago. My chief there was Professor Anton J. Carlson, one of the true giants of physiology. He assigned me the thyroid gland as the subject for my graduate research and doctorate thesis.

33

I was disappointed. As an undergraduate in college, I had done some work in the field of female sex hormones and had hoped to continue with it in graduate school. For some reason, sex seems exciting to young students.

Professor Carlson never knew about my disappointment. This was a time of depression and any job that provided an opportunity to go to graduate school was welcome. The thyroid research was to prove challenging, both immediately and for a lifetime.

One of the duties I was assigned for earning my stipend was teaching a course in endocrinology to medical students. Laboratory animals were used to demonstrate the influence of each of the endocrine glands. A gland would be removed and the results of its removal would be noted over a period of time.

One of the most graphic demonstrations was that in which thyroid glands were removed from baby rabbits. Within two weeks, their fur became dry and began to fall out. After another week, their weights lagged behind those of normal rabbits. As time passed, every cell in their bodies was affected by the lack of thyroid hormone. The thyroidectomized animals suffered repeated infections and died at less than half the normal age. When thyroid was administered to some of the rabbits, there was quick relief for their multiple problems and a seemingly miraculous return to health.

After obtaining my Ph.D., I went on to medical school and completed medical studies in 1937. In practice, like many other physicians, I saw patients who had health problems for which the physical cause was clear. But there were many, too, with complaints that did not fit the usual categories of disease. It wasn't long before I noticed that I was seeing patients whose troubles reminded me of those of rabbits whose thyroid glands had been removed. The troubles were not as extreme but they were reminiscent.

At that time, if a patient had symptoms for which no organic disease explanation could be found, many physicians applied the label "hypochondriac." What else, they thought, could be the problem, since nothing physically was wrong, but an abnormal concern about health and an exaggeration of trivial symptoms? If such labeling did little to help the patient, I am afraid that very often neither does the more sophisticated current term of "psychosomatic complaints."

I had had two tragic experiences within six months after graduating from medical school which I have never forgotten. They have reminded me all through my medical career that there is no justification for a blithe assumption that any complaint for which a physical explanation isn't immediately apparent must be imaginary. A girl in her late teens experienced a variety of peculiar symptoms for which her physicians could find no satisfactory cause. Neither could I, a young neophyte. But when the girl died unexpectedly within a few months, there could be little doubt that she had been suffering from a serious—and undiagnosed—disease.

The second case was that of a young expectant mother who complained of many disturbances including severe headaches. She was checked by many physicians and a neurological study seemed to rule out brain disease. Yet, shortly after she gave birth to her child, she died from a brain tumor. The tumor was very much apparent at autopsy.

These two errors—failures of diagnosis—underscored for me the importance of never making light of a patient's symptoms and history and of making repeated efforts to find a possible physical cause.

Having learned from baby rabbits that thyroid deficiency can produce diverse symptoms, I began early in medical practice to try to screen for possible hypothyroidism any patient whose problems did not fit ordinary disease categories.

But it was no simple matter to do the screening, to determine with any certainty whether a patient had normal thyroid function or was hypothyroid and could benefit from thyroid treatment.

Tests and False Results

It is relatively easy to detect the presence of some disorders—diabetes, for example. Insulin, made in the pancreas, is essential for body metabolism of the sugar glucose. Several tests can reveal diabetes by indicating faulty glucose metabolism. When glucose isn't being used properly, an excess of it can be found in the blood. And because an excess in the blood spills over into the urine, diabetes can be tested for by a simple dipstick procedure—a change of color of specially impregnated paper when it is dipped into a urine sample. One can get an index of kidney function, too, by a simple test to measure certain waste products in the bloodstream.

But thyroid function is another matter. What would be the ideal test for it is not even possible. What we ideally need to measure is the amount of thyroid hormone on the inside of each cell in the body where it controls the rate of oxidation of fuel burning within the cell.

It is obvious, of course, why such a test is impossible. Since there are billions of cells in the body, billions of simultaneous analyses would have to be run and this can't be done even today with computers.

What could be measured—and was—forty years ago was the total oxygen consumption of the body per minute. The test for this—called the basal metabolism test —hopefully provided a check on thyroid function through measurement of the oxygen used when the body is at rest and doing nothing but sustaining itself.

But there were many objections to the basal metabolism test. Basal meant that the body had to be at total rest, free of digestive as well as external activity, and free of tension as well. Exercise, the digestion of food, tension in the muscles, or even worry can increase the rate at which the cells of the body use oxygen.

A true basal state might be measured if a technician were to take all the needed test equipment to the patient's home very early in the morning, stand by until the very moment the patient opened his eyes, and then run the test at once. This, of course, was impractical. So the patient was instructed to get up slowly, dress, make his way to the physician's office through traffic, and there relax for thirty minutes. But the patient's state then is anything but basal.

And the test itself is anything but relaxing. A tight clothespin on the nose and a large rubber breathing tube stuffed in the mouth, or alternatively a tight mask over both nose and mouth, do not make for calm and comfort.

Many errors have been made in basal metabolism tests.

Some verge on being silly. For example, when a student was sent to his family physician for confirmation of a low basal metabolic rate found by a college student health department, the family doctor's test showed the rate to be 40 percent higher than that determined at school. Questioning revealed that the student had been late for his appointment at the doctor's office and, not waiting for the elevator, had run up six flights of stairs for his examination. The doctor had confirmed the influence of exercise.

But many more errors are made because of patient tension and inability to relax thoroughly. I recall a young man who was referred for testing because of suspicion he might have a thyroid problem. During the test, it became obvious that he was not relaxed although he did not move. At the end of the test he was assured that the machine would not bite him and then was told a funny story. A hearty laugh helped him relax and a second test was run within five minutes. The first test had shown +16 percent, indicating above-normal thyroid function; the second test showed −24 percent, indicating markedly below-normal function.

The ability of nervous tension to influence test results is also illustrated by the case of a football player suspected of being hypothyroid. On the morning of his basal metabolism test, he took his temperature before getting out of bed and got a 96.1 reading. While he was resting in the laboratory prior to the test, a thermometer was placed in his mouth and registered 96.4. After the five-minute metabolism test was run, his temperature was taken again and now was 96.9. There had been no exercise or other activity; the excitement of taking the test had been enough to raise his temperature by 0.5 degree and the temperature at the end of the test was 0.8 degree higher than it had been under basal conditions before arising.

It has long been known that the metabolic rate increases as body temperature increases. Hence, the result of this metabolism test, 18 percent, indicating hypothyroidism, was not accurate; the young man was hypothyroid but even more so than the test indicated.

The Search for Other Tests

Many efforts have been made by many investigators to find some means better than the basal metabolism test for checking on thyroid function. For a time, it seemed that determining the cholesterol level in the blood might have some value. An association between high blood cholesterol and thyroid deficiency had been noted.

Yet, when working with students at Armour Tech (now the Illinois Institute of Technology) and at the University of Denver, I checked the cholesterol levels in 500 young men and, as part of the same study, Dr. William B. Brown, Medical Director at Stephens College, Columbia, Missouri, checked the levels in 500 young women, we found that testing for cholesterol could not be relied upon as an indicator of thyroid function in young people. It turned out that the cholesterol level in younger people is often normal regardless of thyroid function and in some older people as well cholesterol level may not be elevated when thyroid function is depressed. It is a fact that when, in anyone, cholesterol level is found to be high, a first wise step is to determine whether there is thyroid deficiency before proceeding to other measures, for often correcting the deficiency will lead to reduction of the cholesterol concentration in the blood. But blood cholesterol level cannot be depended upon as a universal indicator of hypothyroidism.

Many seemingly sophisticated chemical tests have been developed to check on thyroid function and yet they have been no more reliable than the basal metabolism test and have been confusing to many physicians.

Before the turn of the century, it had been determined that the thyroid hormone was a large protein molecule which always contained iodine. Not surprisingly then, the first chemical test for thyroid function sought to measure the amount of protein-bound iodine circulating in the blood. The test is known as the PBI. Unfortunately, iodine from the iodized salt used in the diet can combine with other proteins that have no thyroid hormone activity and the PBI test may mistakenly measure these, failing to show hypothyroidism. Nevertheless, for many years, some otherwise competent physicians swore by the PBI as an accurate index of thyroid function while the rest of us swore at it.

Some years later, the thyroid hormone protein was broken up chemically and yielded a simple iodine-containing material which was found to be active in the body and of some value in treating hypothyroidism. The compound was called thyroxine or T_4 because it contained four atoms of iodine. It seemed to some investigators that thyroxine was *the* thyroid hormone and they proceeded to use it rather than the whole thyroid gland for replacement therapy. Since the PBI would not detect

T4, another test had to be devised. This was called the T4 test and is specific for thyroxine.

But then, still later, another iodine-containing material was isolated from the thyroid protein and, astonishingly enough, proved to be four times more active physiologically than thyroxine. Since it contained three atoms of iodine, it was called triiodothyronine or T3. Its advent may have embarrassed those who had insisted that T4 was *the* thyroid hormone. In any case, with T3 now on the scene, a new test was called for and there followed the development of a T3 test. Now the T3 test would detect T3 but not T4; the T4 test would detect only T4, not T3; and the PBI would detect neither.

Many other tests aimed at trying to evaluate thyroid function have been developed over the years. Their variety is dazzling; their interpretation difficult. To mention just one here, when a small cocktail containing radioactive iodine is swallowed, the iodine tends to be attracted to the thyroid gland, and the amount of the iodine retained by the gland can be determined. This, hopefully, provides some information about thyroid gland function. But the test is expensive, requires two trips by the patient to the radiation laboratory, and the results are often less informative than they should be.

The efforts through the various tests to measure thyroid activity by determining the amount of hormone stored in the gland or alternatively the amount present in the bloodstream fail to do what really counts: provide an indication of the amount of thyroid hormone available and being used within cells throughout the body. They are somewhat akin to trying to get an idea of a thrifty man's spending habits from the amount of money in his wallet or the size of his bank account. The amounts of money in wallet or bank account, like tests for the amount of hormone in gland or bloodstream, tell us nothing about how much is being spent.

A Clue to a Simple Test

Some of the earliest studies of hypothyroid patients, which had been done in England, noted that they ran temperatures below the normal range. This was understandable. Under any circumstances, the amount of heat produced must, of course, depend upon the amount of fuel burned. Body heat depends upon the amount of foodstuffs burned. The body thermostat of a thyroid-deficient person may call for more heat, but thyroid hormone is essential for the oxidation or burning of fuel in the body, and in the thyroid-deficient person body temperature falls below normal because of inadequate oxidation. On the other hand, if too much thyroid hormone is circulating, so much heat is produced that the thermostat cannot control the temperature precisely and a low-grade fever results.

In the early years of my medical practice, I ran many basal metabolism tests and it was always necessary to take a patient's temperature as a precaution before attempting to administer a test. For if any infection was present, metabolism would be higher because of the elevated temperature and the test would not be accurate.

Particularly at the University of Denver, in the course of performing basal metabolism tests on many hundreds of students, I noted the consistency with which those with low metabolic rates as shown by the basal metabolism test also had lower-than-normal temperatures.

The thought occurred that perhaps basal temperature might be as accurate as basal metabolism as a test for thyroid function. Perhaps it might even be more so. The patient could take his own temperature immediately upon awakening in the morning before engaging in any activity or eating anything and there would be no inconvenience or expense.

I decided to try to find out and for my first, early attempts, I instructed patients to follow a simple procedure: Place a thermometer, well-shaken down, by the bedside at night upon retiring. Upon awakening in the morning, the very first thing they were to do, before stirring from bed, was to reach out for the thermometer, place it in the mouth, and leave it there for ten minutes by the clock while resting quietly.

In August 1942, I could report in *The Journal of the American Medical Association* on a study with one thousand college students whose basal temperatures were taken and who also received basal metabolism tests. The study indicated that a subnormal body temperature is a better index of hypothyroidism and the need for thyroid treatment than the basal metabolic rate.

Among the patients were some with neurasthenia, chronic nervous exhaustion, arthritis, and other problems not generally considered to have anything to do with low thyroid function. Yet the initial low basal temperature and the improvement seen when the temperature was raised by thyroid therapy suggested that hypothyroidism might well be a factor of some importance in such problems and further studies of the possibility seemed warranted.

It was also possible to note in the report that among other patients with subnormal basal temperature, a rise of the temperature with thyroid therapy led to perceptible improvement in performance, whether in the classroom, or the athletic field, or in industry.

The basal body temperature test, moreover, apparently could set straight erroneous diagnoses, as in the case of a twenty-two-year-old woman who had been very nervous and markedly underweight for several years and suffered from palpitations, high blood pressure, a fast pulse rate of 110, and tremor of the hands. Prior to entering the university, her basal metabolic rate had been found to be +18 and she had been advised to have a thyroidectomy as a means of relieving her seeming *hyper*thyroidism, or overfunctioning of the thyroid. She had refused the operation.

Her body temperature was 97.6. Her basal metabolic rate, when she was now tested again, was +8 percent. But it was obvious during the basal metabolic rate test that she was not relaxed. She was then given a mild sedative to be taken several times a day for the next week after which the basal metabolism test was repeated. Now the result was −8 percent, and the basal metabolism test was showing what the subnormal body temperature had already indicated—that this was a young woman not with an *over*active but rather with an *under*active thyroid.

She was started on a small dose of thyroid. Over a period of sixty days, as her body temperature gradually rose in response to the thyroid, her blood pressure fell to normal, her pulse rate came down to 84, her nervousness and her hand tremor improved.

This simple technique of measuring basal body temperature as a guide to determining thyroid function and permitting proper treatment when necessary did not appeal to the medical profession. Apparently some physicians had reservations about a test which might permit patients to arrive at their own diagnoses. Perhaps some had reservations because the test involved no fee.

Refining the Test

Service in the armed forces during World War II interrupted for a time my work on basal temperature, but then provided an opportunity to refine the test by determining at which location the basal temperature is best taken.

Whenever there is a local infection or inflammation, the temperature in that area of the body is elevated. One of the most common infections is sinusitis which will raise the temperature in the mouth and in so doing may make an under-the-tongue thermometer reading misleading.

During the war, I was stationed at a military base in Kingman, Arizona. Dr. Joseph Ehrlich, who was stationed at another military base, joined me in a study in which we determined simultaneously the oral, rectal, and armpit temperatures of one thousand soldiers. These lonesome men were only too glad to be disturbed for ten minutes just prior to reveille in return for some personal attention.

Dr. Ehrlich and I found that in the absence of oral

infection, the temperatures of the mouth and of the armpit were almost identical when thermometers were left in place for ten minutes. The rectal temperature averaged almost a degree higher than either oral or armpit temperature.

Thus, it seemed that axillary, or underarm, temperature might serve as a simple guide to determining low thyroid function and the need for thyroid therapy. And over the past thirty years, it has served as such. In that time, based on many thousands of readings, it has been established that normal values for underarm temperature are in the range of 97.8 to 98.2 degrees Fahrenheit. A temperature below 97.8 indicated hypothyroidism; one above 98.2, hyperthyroidism. And, when thyroid therapy is indicated for low thyroid function, the simple test can be used to monitor the therapy. As low temperature rises with thyroid treatment, the symptoms associated with hypothyroidism will disappear. And there is no risk of excessive thyroid dosage as long as basal temperature does not exceed 98.2.

The basal temperature is not a perfect test for thyroid function. There are conditions other than hypothyroidism that may produce a low reading—for example, starvation, pituitary gland deficiency, or adrenal gland deficiency. But starvation is certainly not difficult to rule out—and some thyroid is frequently indicated, anyhow, for the other conditions.

More information often can be brought to the physician with only the aid of an ordinary thermometer than can be obtained with all other thyroid function tests combined.

Just as the British were the first to recognize thyroid deficiency, the first to synthesize the thyroid hormone thyroxin, the first to recognize a second active compound, T3, and the first in many other areas of thyroid study and treatment, so were they the first to compare various thyroid diagnostic tests. It was a British investigator who, in 1960, reported extensive studies on one hundred proven cases of thyroid deficiency. In these one hundred patients, everyone with definite hypothyroidism, the basal metabolism test was correct in diagnosing only 77 percent—and there was no significant difference in diagnostic accuracy between the basal metabolism and other tests such as the PBI, thyroxin, and cholesterol. A whole battery of such tests could still miss about twenty cases of hypothyroidism out of one hundred.

Although the basal temperature test is not 100 percent specific for thyroid function, the simple procedure is remarkably successful in uncovering hypothyroidism. Its results most often fit well with patients' symptoms.

Taking the Test

The basal temperature can be taken by a man on any given day. Not so for a woman. During the menstrual years, temperature fluctuates during the cycle, as every woman knows. It is highest shortly before the start of the menstrual flow and lowest at the time of ovulation. During a woman's menstrual years, then, the temperature curve is such that basal temperature is best measured on the second and third days of the period after flow starts. Before the menarche or after the menopause, the basal temperature may be taken on any day.

When no other reason can be found, no clear-cut diagnosis made, to explain the presence of a symptom or a whole complex of symptoms, it is worthwhile taking a thermometer to bed with you. Shake it down well and place it on the night stand. Immediately upon awakening in the morning, place the thermometer snugly in the armpit for ten minutes by the clock. A reading below the normal range of 97.8 to 98.2 strongly suggests low thyroid function. If the reading is above the normal range, one must be suspicious of some infection or an overactive thyroid gland.

For small children who are likely to resist being quiet for ten minutes, more accurate readings often can be obtained by taking the temperature rectally for two minutes. The normal range of rectal temperature is about one degree higher than that of the armpit—98.8 to 99.2.

A True Picture of Low Thyroid

Over the past four decades there have been reports from discerning physicians that hypothyroidism is commonly unrecognized—and if part of the reason has been the confusion of tests for the condition, another important part has been confusion over the condition itself.

As far back as 1933, Dr. O.P. Kimball, after a ten-year study—five years of it carried out at the famed Cleveland Clinic and five years in private practice—was reporting that "In the practice of medicine today no more important condition is encountered or so often unrecognized as such, as hypothyroidism."

And Dr. Kimball went on to note that a cardinal reason for this was a theory that hypothyroidism couldn't exist without myxedema. On the very face of it, the theory was ridiculous, presupposing as it did that there couldn't be milder degrees of hypothyroidism, only a failure of the thyroid gland so great that it produced extreme symptoms. Yet that was the theory that he had been taught as a medical student, Dr. Kimball noted, and went on to add: "Just why this teaching should persist now in the face of all the experimental evidence to the contrary is hard to understand."

There was to be more experimental evidence to the contrary in the years that followed—and still the theory persisted. Half a dozen years after Dr. Kimball published his report, Dr. G.K. Wharton of the University of Western Ontario published another which decried essentially the same thing: "Many patients who could be helped by thyroid treatment are not recognized as hypothyroid. Cretinism and myxedema are the textbook examples of the hypofunctioning thyroid gland. Very little has been written about the milder degrees and the atypical forms of deficient thyroid activity. Hypothyroidism in a mild or masked form differs so greatly from myxedema and cretinism that constant alertness for its many and varied manifestations is demanded."

And still many years later, Dr. Arnold Jackson was trying to call the attention of the medical profession, in a report in *The Journal of the American Medical Association,* to the fact that "Hypothyroidism is the most frequent chronic affliction and at the same time the most often overlooked condition affecting persons residing in the Middle West. This statement is based upon an experience of thirty-seven years in diagnosing and treating thousands of these cases seen at the Mayo and Jackson clinics."

I would modify Dr. Jackson's statement only to the extent that hypothyroidism remains the most frequent and often overlooked chronic condition affecting people residing all over the United States as they have spread out from the United States goiter belt and from goiter belts abroad and taken up residence all over the country.

As the following chapters will show, hypothyroidism of the mild to moderate kind—far short of the kind that leads to cretinism or myxedema—can be and very often is responsible for a very wide range of health problems and hazards, and its recognition and proper treatment can have profoundly beneficial consequences.

4

The Thyroid and Fatigue

NOT LONG AGO, after a national magazine published an article on some of the problems associated with low thyroid function and described the basal temperature test, a sixty-six-year-old woman hopefully came to see me from a considerable distance.

Her major complaint was fatigue. For much of her life, she told me, she had felt that she lacked ordinary pep. She had gotten along fairly well in her younger years but it had seemed to her that she had had to push herself hard to overcome a kind of inertia that stemmed from lack of a normal amount of energy. She had always needed nine or ten hours of sleep. She was a heavy coffee drinker, using it to try to pep herself up.

At various times, she had sought medical help for the fatigue—and there had been efforts to help. "Tonics" had been prescribed many years before and when, during her menstrual years, there had been some evidence of at least slight anemia, there had been treatment for that. But the fatigue had persisted.

It had become worse in recent years. Several years ago, she had checked into a major private clinic for thorough study. When nothing physical could be found to explain her fatigue, the suggestion was that perhaps a psychiatrist could help. Instead, she had gone to a West Coast university hospital where again many tests failed to pinpoint any physical cause and again it was suggested that a psychiatrist might help. She then did consult a psychiatrist who, after several sessions, told her quite frankly that he didn't know what was causing her problem but he did feel certain that it was not a psychiatric problem.

When I saw her, she had come armed with the clinic and hospital records—and with a temperature record. She had taken her basal temperature at home a dozen times. It was consistently low. She was started on a small dose of thyroid. It was increased gradually until her basal temperature rose. As it did so, her abnormal fatigue disappeared.

There is nothing at all unusual about her case. A low energy level with easy fatigability can have other causes, certainly. It is, however, a common problem of the hypothyroid and has long been known to be. Some studies have shown it to be a major complaint in as many as 98 percent of all patients found to be hypothyroid by basal metabolism, PBI, and other standard tests.

But many of the fatigued do not receive such tests; the possibility of hypothyroidism goes unsuspected. And many who have had the tests have, in effect, "failed" them—or, more accurately, the tests have failed them, indicating normal thyroid function when it hasn't been normal at all.

Repeatedly, I see patients who have suffered for long periods with excessive fatigue and whose suffering has been needless.

The Repercussions of Fatigue

A low energy level can take a mental and emotional as well as physical toll—and can do so at any age. In childhood and youth, it may be responsible for difficulties in school and in parent-child relationships, and sometimes for delinquent behavior.

Children, of course, like to be praised. They work hard for rewards. The child who seemingly is not interested in making any effort, who seems just "pure lazy," may not be pure lazy at all and may be fully as interested in making efforts as any other child but is handicapped by a lack of sufficient energy to meet daily challenges.

Many of these handicapped youngsters try hard only to be frustrated. Some become school dropouts and may even resort to petty crimes and, in doing so, may achieve some "success" for the first time in their lives. Some turn to drugs as an escape from reality.

A seventeen-year-old I saw recently had complained for years of being tired. He came from an excellent family of some means and he, like his brothers and sisters, was well provided for. But he could not function as did his siblings. Even after a prolonged night's sleep, he had difficulty getting up in the morning. In school, he was unable to think clearly and to concentrate, and repeatedly failed.

He dropped out, tried work, but lost job after job because of lateness. He began to run with the wrong crowd, took to hard drugs, had an encounter with the law. Fortunately, in the sense of better late rather than never, his fatigue (and the effects of it) were found to be associated with a subnormal basal temperature and within three months after therapy was begun he was enrolled in a rehabilitation program and in school again, very much interested now in trying, and better able to make something of his life.

Recently, I saw an eight-year-old victim of fatigue. The child was affected to the point where he refused to go out and play with other children. In school, his work was poor and his teachers were convinced he was not living up to his innate capabilities. For a time, his parents thought he was simply a lazy child. Then, considering the possibility that he might be emotionally ill, they entertained the idea of seeking psychiatric help. But they decided that they would try, at least one more time, to get medical help. The child's thyroid function, never even tested for before, was decidedly low; his response to thyroid therapy was gratifying.

Several years ago, a friend of our family mentioned her problem one night while having dinner with us. Her problem was an eighteen-year-old son, a senior in high school, a big fellow, 6'3", 200 pounds, and a basketball player of some ability. What bothered her about the boy was his attitude at home: he was withdrawn, had little to do with the family, refused to keep his room reasonably neat and orderly. His school work, too, it seemed to her, was not what it should be. In talking with her, I discovered, too, that although he was one of the high school basketball team's stars, he had to have frequent rest intervals during a game, playing only for short periods at a time.

Here was another low thyroid function victim. He expended as much energy as he could muster at what he liked best of all—basketball. He had little left for school work, for interacting with the family, for carrying out routine chores. His response, too, on thyroid therapy was gratifying.

Like that eighteen-year-old, many adults with low thyroid function, although handicapped by inadequate energy, are not entirely defeated by it. Many are successful in their work—but at a price. All of their small store of vitality is used up in accomplishing what they most want to accomplish, leaving little or none for other aspects of life. And many, aware of how much they are missing, may experience bouts of anxiety or depression. Often, too, their fatigue may lead to physical complaints, among which, as we shall see later, headache is a common one.

Causes

Fatigue is a normal result of intense physical exertion, emotional stress, or lack of rest. It is the body's signaling of a need to slow down, relax, get more sleep and rest.

Fatigue that is not relieved by rest has another origin. It may be a symptom of any of a considerable number of possible problems, including, of course, poor living habits. Even sedentary living, with insufficient physical activity, may sometimes be the reason for undue fatigue.

It has been estimated that with maximum effort, the human body can generate as much as 14 horsepower; at rest, it generates only 0.1 horsepower. And in some of those who lead sedentary lives, there is a degree of muscular atrophy, or wasting away, so that they become undermuscled for their weight and may lack the strength and endurance needed even for sedentary work. It may be, too, that in some who lead sedentary existences, the unused horsepower in effect goes into building up of tension, and the tension then becomes a factor in producing fatigue and sometimes other complaints as well.

Physicians have reported many cases like that of a man in his midthirties who had progressed well in his career and should have been happy and at the height of his capacity. Instead, he complained of chronic fatigue, sleeping difficulties, growing inability to concentrate effectively and handle his work almost effortlessly as he once had done. When, in his case, no medication was prescribed but rather a program of activity, of regular exercise beginning easily and progressing gradually, a marked change occurred within a few months. Activity reinvigorated him.

Sometimes, fatigue can be psychologic in origin. Tiredness and loss of interest in one's work can stem from boredom. And if this is really the case, if there is certainty that nothing is wrong physically, varying daily activities as much as possible and seeking new interests and new ways to spend leisure time may do much to relieve the fatigue by overcoming the boredom.

Sometimes, a state of abnormal fatigue may be brought on by emotional problems which, if long continued, may lead to mental and physical exhaustion. But while emotional problems can be capable of producing such exhaustion, it must not be assumed, even when they are clearly present, that they are doing so until the possibility of a physical cause has been carefully considered.

Fatigue is associated with a wide variety of diseases. They include tuberculosis, heart ailments, diabetes, and cancer, for example. They also include anemia and thyroid disorder—and, as we shall now see, these two can be associated.

Anemia

A common idea is that very often the reason for chronic fatigue is anemia and that the reason for the anemia is "iron-poor" blood or vitamin deficiency, or both.

That anemia is repsonsible for much undue tiredness is true, but that it is all a matter of lack of iron or of vitamins is not true. What too often goes unappreciated is the role of thyroid deficiency in producing anemia, in contributing to its effects, and even in producing anemialike states.

Anemia means a deficiency in either the quantity or quality of blood. Usually the term refers to a decrease in the number of red blood cells (erythrocytes) or a reduction in hemoglobin.

Blood normally contains about five million red cells per cubic millimeter. These cells are packed with hemoglobin, the pigment which gives blood its red color, and which also has an affinity for oxygen. It is hemoglobin which serves the vital function of picking up and combining with oxygen in the lungs and then transporting it and releasing it to all tissues of the body. On the average, each 100 cubic centimeters of blood contains 15 grams of hemoglobin so that there is about one-half ounce of hemoglobin for every 3½ ounces of blood.

Since the ability of the blood to carry oxygen depends upon an adequate number of red cells and adequate hemoglobin in each of them, anemia of some degree develops when either is reduced.

With mild degrees of anemia, symptoms may be vague and slight, perhaps only a feeling of some reduction in energy and a tendency to become fatigued more often and more easily. With more severe anemia, the fatigue may become oppressive. In still more severe anemia, exertion may cause shortness of breath, some pounding of the heart, and a more rapid pulse rate. With very severe anemia, there may be fainting spells, dizziness, headaches, ringing in the ears, loss of appetite, and sometimes swelling of the ankles. It is only with moderate or severe anemia, not mild, that a patient usually looks pale, and the pallor usually is best detected in the palms of the hands and the fingernails.

It has been said that just one-fifth of an ounce of iron stands between us and suffocation. For iron goes into the making of hemoglobin, and anemia can result when a deficiency of iron leads to a deficiency of hemoglobin.

Iron deficiency can stem from chronic loss of blood. In women, the deficiency may result from excess menstrual flow; in men, from the slow bleeding of a peptic ulcer; in both sexes, from hemorrhoids or piles. There are other possible causes: hiatus hernia, large doses of aspirin or aspirin-related compounds, tumors of stomach or intestine which may bleed, hookworm infestation. Failure to take in enough iron in the diet—as when a person lives on tea and toast or coffee and doughnuts or goes on a prolonged fad diet—can produce iron deficiency.

But iron may be plentiful—and so may vitamins and other essentials—and yet anemia may develop when not enough red blood cells are produced.

Years ago, at one of the regular Monday afternoon physiology seminars at the University of Chicago, I heard an enlightening presentation of a rather remarkable bit of research. Red blood cells are manufactured in the bone marrow, the soft, spongelike material in the cavities of bones. A study had been done on the effect of the temperature of the bone marrow on the formation of red cells. It had long been known that marrow differs at different sites in bone. In bone in the upper part of the arms and legs, the marrow is red and forms blood cells, but in the lower reaches of the extremities, the marrow color is white and no blood is formed.

In the study, careful electrical measurements of temperature along bone revealed a drop in temperature toward the lower reaches of the extremities. And the temperature effect on color of marrow and red cell formation was demonstrated by an ingenious experiment with the tail of a white rat. All of the marrow in the rat's tail was white and formed no blood. The tip of the tail was inserted into the rat's belly through a surgical opening and sutured there where the temperature was higher. Shortly, the very tip of the tail, now at higher temperature within the belly, began to form blood while the rest of the tail, outside the belly and at lower temperature, continued to have white marrow and form no blood.

Thus, it would seem that a subnormal temperature which is characteristic of low thyroid function can contribute to anemia by its effects on blood cell production in the bone marrow. And the elevation of subnormal temperature to normal by thyroid therapy may help to explain the absence of chronic anemia in thousands of patients I have seen over past thirty-five years whose hypothyroidism has been corrected, including many who previously had been diagnosed as anemic.

Another Factor

The hypothyroid patient may experience effects like those produced by anemia, including undue fatigue, for another reason. Thyroid deficiency tends to reduce the strength of the heartbeat, and the amount of blood pumped out to the body with each beat is reduced.

In severe hypothyroidism, studies have shown that the blood circulating per minute through the body may be reduced by as much as 40 percent, thus the effective oxygen-carrying capacity of the blood is only 60 percent of normal. In milder cases of reduced thyroid function, the reduction in circulation is, of course, not nearly that severe. Yet even mild reduction of circulation, despite the presence of adequate hemoglobin and adequate red cells, can mean that less than normal amounts of oxygen are reaching the tissues which are always anemic to a degree.

Any person with hypothyroid fatigue fights an uphill battle—getting physically tired sooner and taking longer to recuperate. That person is more prone to mental as well as physical fatigue, and, even after extended rest, the brain, like the rest of the body, gets something less than adequate circulation and this is no aid to thought processes.

The mental fatigue, if severe enough, can be much like that of the battle fatigue suffered by soldiers during prolonged front-line duty in war. And daily life for a hypothyroid person might well seem to the normal individual to be almost the equivalent of combat duty.

Yet this is needless. I don't for one moment mean to imply that thyroid therapy is a panacea. But when thyroid function is low, when subnormal basal temperature indicates so, and when this is so in a person with low energy reserve and chronic fatigue, physical or mental, there is every likelihood that thyroid therapy can produce a remarkable change.

It can frequently produce striking benefits, too, when fatigue and the impaired circulation that contributes to it lead to an accumulation of fluid in the tissues and, as we shall see in the next chapter, to an abnormal allotment of headaches.

5

Migraine
and Other Headaches

FOR A TIME not long after I graduated from medical
school, I shared an office in Chicago with a physician who
suffered from migraine headaches. Migraine often tends
to run in families and his mother had been a victim. His
own migraine had begun at an early age. He could remember vividly that as a child whenever the circus came
to town or he became overly excited about anything else,
or unduly tired, he would develop a severe headache.

Throughout his career, which was a brilliant one—he
was one of Chicago's most distinguished internists—he
was aware that he tended to become fatigued easily and
that when he became overly fatigued or overly involved
emotionally, he would almost invariably have a migraine
attack that would incapacitate him for two or three days.

When I met him, his migraine had taken a turn for the
worse. He was at the height of his career, was often called

upon to travel long distances for consultations. The trips, on top of his already extremely busy local practice, were fatiguing. He was having marital problems and there was additional intense stress in his life because of some rather large investments which had gone sour.

His migraine attacks were coming more and more often and their severity was increasing. Secretly, he was concerned that something new had been added: that, conceivably, a brain tumor might have developed and could be responsible for aggravating his lifelong headache problem.

One day, I got up nerve enough to corner him and insist that something must be done about the headaches; that either he go to a clinic for study or let me try to check into the problem. He decided that he would let me try to help but insisted that, in order to keep office employees from knowing about it, I must come to his home.

I called at his home early one morning, was admitted by his wife, and found him still in bed. While he remained in bed, I took his temperature and found it low. His pulse rate also was low: 44. I examined him thoroughly and drew blood for laboratory tests. The tests revealed nothing, no abnormality.

The low temperature and the low pulse rate indicated low thyroid function and I suggested that we should certainly do something about that. He agreed to thyroid therapy but had no faith that this would do anything for his headaches. Nor, in fact, did I at the time. Yet, within a few weeks, both of us were agreeably surprised. Even as he began to feel less tired as the result of the thyroid therapy, his headaches began to diminish in intensity and frequency. Over a period of several months, as he became increasingly vigorous, his migraine attacks diminished almost to the vanishing point, appearing only when he unwisely allowed himself to be caught up in social activities to the point where he cut short his sleep for several nights in a row.

This experience started me on a new approach to migraine. Of the many theories advanced to try to explain the mechanism of headache, raised pressure within the brain appeared to be the most plausible. I was aware of the theory. I also became aware as I worked with migraine patients that fatigue seemed to play an important role in initiating their attacks. Almost invariably, migraine victims, upon reflection, would indicate that their attacks came on when they were very tired. They also indicated, when questioned, that as their attacks came on, they often had to loosen their shoelaces because they felt their shoes becoming tight. Many of the women victims recalled that they had difficulty removing wedding rings during a siege. And they added that the only thing they could do about their migraine attacks was to go to bed and rest.

Every migraine patient coming my way was carefully studied. A complete medical history was taken, a thorough physical examination was carried out, and laboratory tests were performed. In every case, too, basal temperature was taken. And in virtually every case, there was evidence of low thyroid function. So thyroid medication was used. Within thirty days after thyroid therapy was started, a marked decrease in both frequency and severity of migraine was the rule. Of the first 100 migraine patients so studied and treated, 95 benefitted.

Why? Fatigue can produce changes in the body. Waste products accumulate. Blood vessels become dilated. With prolonged fatigue, tissues swell. Swelling of the feet is quite common during excessive fatigue. It seems reasonable to suppose that other tissues as well swell and that the brain is not exempt from such swelling which would cause undue pressure in the rigid cranium with pain resulting.

When the fatigue is associated with low thyroid function, thyroid therapy raises the threshold to fatigue and in so doing may reduce the frequency and severity of headaches.

Certainly, low thyroid function is not the cause of every case of migraine. There may be other factors —allergy, for example—and some migraine victims may benefit if an offending agent can be identified and then eliminated.

But my experience convinces me that every patient suffering from migraine—or from other severe, recurring headaches—deserves a study in which basal temperature is checked.

I recall an interesting case encountered during World War II when a thirty-nine-year-old cousin of my wife visited us not long after being drafted into the army. His mother had had migraine and as a child he had shown some propensity to headaches although at that time they apparently weren't migrainous or "sick headaches."

In his late teens, however, he developed full-fledged migraine. His father, a dentist, had insisted that his son must follow in his footsteps. But the son could not drive himself toward dentistry and there was conflict for years which might have been blamed for the headaches by those inclined to believe that they have a psychosomatic origin.

At the university he had attended, he had been

thoroughly investigated not only by physicians of the student health service but also by others on the faculty of the medical school there and by physicians at a well-known private clinic. The headaches went on.

After college, he had entered upon a literary career and, despite his migraine episodes, was doing well. He had married just a few months before being drafted. It was something of a wrench to go into the army. When I first saw him, he had just left his bride and was headed overseas for duty with a truck driving unit and not looking forward to the assignment.

He was placed on thyroid therapy when, during his visit with us, I found his thyroid function low. He served overseas, not happily but with much less disability from migraine than in previous years. After the war, he resumed a distinguished career as an editor; he still takes his thyroid to avoid migraine.

Other Headaches

It isn't only migraine to which low thyroid function may contribute. Tension headaches, which are much more common than migraine and may account for about 70 percent of all headaches, may stem from the low threshold to fatigue and to stress that so often accompanies low thyroid function.

When I was associated with the medical services at both the Armour Institute of Technology and the University of Denver, I saw many students with relatively mild hypothyroidism who got along fairly well under ordinary circumstances. Their energy wasn't all it should have been; they tended to become fatigued more easily than other people of their age; they had a few more headaches than the normal allotment.

But at examination times when they were under stress, cramming hard and cutting back on sleep, they were hit by severe headaches and many failed to do well on their exams. Other students went through the same process of cramming but were not similarly affected because their thresholds for fatigue were much higher. Thyroid treatment helped many of these low thyroid young people. It has done the same for many hundreds of patients of all ages.

Again, I want to emphasize that headaches can have many causes, including infectious diseases, liver and gall bladder disturbances, high blood pressure, low blood sugar, and much more. Any physician confronted with a patient with chronic severe headaches has to consider many possibilities.

It is important that low thyroid function be considered as one possibility. If the basal temperature is found to be low, and if there is no other immediately obvious cause, the likelihood is great that thyroid therapy will help the headaches.

6

The Thyroid in Emotional and Behavioral Problems

SHE WAS A THIRTY-YEAR-OLD housewife and mother of three children, aged seven, eight, and nine, and her history was one of repeated mental depression. Her "blue" feelings had begun with her first pregnancy and had become so intense in the midst of it that it was thought necessary to resort to electroshock therapy.

There was a return of the depression during each of her subsequent pregnancies, a little less intense, and antidepressant medication was used. But then subsequently she had required institutionalization for treatment on two occasions, each time seeming to improve but then relapsing again.

When I first saw her in 1971, she was again seriously depressed, apathetic, withdrawn, unable to sleep, unable to care for her children. Both her father and her brother were patients of mine. Both were hypothyroid and under treatment and although neither had had emotional or behavioral disturbances associated with their low thyroid function, her father insisted that it could do no harm to check her for it, and brought her to see me.

She *was* hypothyroid. Her basal temperature was well below normal. After six weeks on thyroid therapy which, as always, began with very small dosages, she began to show some improvement, becoming less apathetic and withdrawn, able to sleep better. As we gradually adjusted her thyroid dosage upward to fully compensate for her hypothyroidism, she continued to improve. Within six months, she was entirely out of her depression and on continued thyroid therapy remains so.

There is nothing new in the fact that hypothyroidism can have mental and emotional effects. This is one of the oldest known facts about the condition. Those effects may be the only strikingly apparent symptoms associated with low thyroid function or may be present along with many others. Yet very often no consideration may be given to the thyroid.

One patient I saw not long ago is a thirty-nine-year-old psychologist who, almost all of his life, had been in poor physical health and then, through much of his adult life, had suffered from emotional difficulties. He could remember his aunt applying potato poultices to his head when he was five years old because of his severe, recurrent headaches. He had been an easily fatigued child and one who suffered repeatedly from upper respiratory infections often complicated by earaches and on one occasion a ruptured eardrum. He had a severe bout of pneumonia as a child and another when he was thirty-five.

He was married at the age of eighteen and had one son. He was divorced by his wife after seventeen years of marriage because of his chronic illness and inability to hold a job. At the age of twenty-five, he had become so severely depressed that he had contemplated suicide. There had been psychiatric treatment for the depression and there had been repeated studies seeking to determine the cause of his general ill health. At one point, after a minor automobile accident which seemed to make his headaches worse, he had been hospitalized for two months during which an almost endless series of tests produced only negative results. And since then he had been unable to work at all.

His whole history, certainly the physical ill health, suggested that he might be hypothyroid and I was hardly surprised when his basal temperature proved to be 96 degrees. He is responding to thyroid therapy. The headaches have diminished greatly; he reports feeling more vigorous than ever before in his life; his depressed mood seems to be completely lifted; he has recently found a new job.

It is often said that this is an age of anxiety; that emotional disorders are rife; that many, even most of the patients physicians see, have physical disorders that stem from emotional difficulties, that are psychosomatic in nature.

But I wonder. I have no doubt that there are many psychosomatic problems and that many may stem from emotional disturbances that have nothing to do with the thyroid. But I have no doubt, too, that many of the emotional disturbances have very much to do with thyroid function and that many people are suffering needlessly for failure to recognize that fact.

The First One Hundred

It wasn't very long after hypothyroidism was first identified in England in 1873 that its ability to affect the mind and emotions was recognized. In 1888, a British commission, which had been formed five years before to look into this strange condition called myxedema, the name first applied to hypothyroidism, issued its report on a study of one hundred cases.

All of the myxedematous patients, the commission noted, were slow in thought and response, suffered from poor memory, and almost half had delusions, hallucinations, or frank insanity. Nervousness and irritability were common.

Shortly after the turn of the century, Dr. G.R. Murray, a British physician who was the first to treat myxedema successfully, produced his monumental work, *A System of Medicine,* in which he went into detail on how the symptoms of the condition developed. Languor or listless indolence was often the first to appear, and ordinary daily tasks that previously had been performed without conscious effort became irksome. Sensitivity to cold often followed.

Early in the disease, Dr. Murray found, there might sometimes be auditory or visual hallucinations. (I was to remember this when years ago I saw a thirteen-year-old girl who was helping her destitute family by cleaning rooms part-time in a motel and who, while working, would hear voices. I had never before been confronted with a child suffering from hallucinations but, recalling Murray's association of them with myxedema, I tested the girl for thyroid function and, finding it low, placed her on thyroid therapy. The hallucinations stopped only to return some months later when she lapsed in therapy. Starting thyroid again solved the hallucination problem.)

Dr. Murray reported that all sufferers from severe hypothyroidism showed mental hebetude; they were slow in comprehending a new subject or in following any new line of thought. About one-fourth of them showed a tendency to spend an unusual amount of time at simple tasks and could take as much as an hour to dress or eat a simple meal.

Irritability was common. Many preferred seclusion, wanting nothing to do with others. Acute or chronic mania, melancholia or dementia might develop unless treatment was started early. As Murray pointed out in 1908, thyroid therapy could relieve all of the mental disturbances of these myxedematous, severely hypo-thyroid patients.

Interestingly enough, among the other symptoms that sometimes developed in myxedema, Murray noted, was a fearful suspicion of others. Many years later, in 1949, *The British Medical Journal* carried a report on a medical officer in the British army who had become suspicious that everyone was trying to poison him. He refused to eat. Fortunately, he was thoroughly studied, found to have hypothyroidism, and his psychiatric problems disappeared completely on thyroid therapy. He was returned to duty and functioned well until his tour of army duty was over and he returned to civilian life. He neglected his therapy after discharge and again became psychotic. Resumption of thyroid therapy again restored sanity.

Other Demonstrations

The marked effect of the thyroid gland on behavior, even the most fundamental behavior, has been shown in animals. When the thyroid glands of a pregnant bitch and her unborn puppies are destroyed by use of radioactive iodine, the puppies at birth have lost the basic inherited reflex for nursing and have to be fed artificially.

It has been observed in the past that a human mother with severe hypothyroidism may give birth to a baby doomed to developmental failure and mental retardation.

Physicians before the turn of the century were well aware of the role of thyroid deficiency in mental disturbances although somehow this information has faded from medical teaching. For one thing, the awareness came from experience with patients after the removal of huge goiters that had threatened to suffocate them by compressing the windpipe. The surgery was a desperate measure at a time when thyroid replacement therapy was not available. It was resorted to as possibly the lesser of two evils.

Severe behavioral as well as other changes could follow the removal of the thyroid gland with resulting hypothyroidism. One of the cases reported in the medical literature back then was that of a ten-year-old boy. Six months after thyroid removal, there was what was called a "marked psychical change." The child, once bright and lively, had become quiet and retiring. His growth stopped. The expression on his face became that of an idiot. His hair became sparse. His speech was slow and labored, his heart action weak, and he had difficulty walking even short distances.

He could learn nothing in school and left at age fourteen. Unable to work in the fields because of weakness, he took up knitting, but even that became too much of a chore. He became incapable of thinking. His visual and auditory powers deteriorated. He died at age twenty-eight in a coma, possibly due to liver failure.

I have seen, in both children and adults, many diverse types of behavioral manifestations associated with hypothyroidism of lesser degree.

Some Child Patients

I recall a ten-year-old boy who began to experience nightmarish dreams and would scream for long periods before his parents could get him awake enough to reassure him that he was only having a dream. The terrifying dreams kept increasing in frequency until they were occurring almost nightly and sometimes several times a night. The only definite physical finding in the child was a subnormal basal temperature. On thyroid therapy, the dreams ceased.

As mentioned previously, one of the remarkable features of hypothyroidism is that it may produce seemingly paradoxical effects—both physically and mentally. On the one hand, a marked deficiency occurring at an early age may lead to growth failure and dwarfism; yet, on the other hand, a minor deficiency not only may allow growth to proceed at a normal rate but to be accelerated and extended, producing a seven-footer.

Similarly, there are diverse and seemingly paradoxical effects on energy and behavior. The ten-year-old boy mentioned previously, whose thyroid was removed, became physically and mentally lethargic. Some children with lesser degrees of hypothyroidism are affected in much the same way but to a lesser extent. On the other hand, some hypothyroid children are hyperactive. Their seemingly endless energy might make one think that they have too much rather than too little thyroid activity.

One twelve-year-old boy was so hyperactive and restless that he had been placed in a special school. When his family brought him to see me, he had, within two minutes after entering my office, touched everything in the waiting room and was ready to explore the rest of the building. He lacked normal muscular coordination, a characteristic of many hypothyroid children. He was placed on thyroid therapy with gratifying results. The following year, he was attending regular school, and had become a quiet, studious fellow able to compete with his peers.

Other characteristics are often shared by hypothyroid children and those who, without regard to thyroid function, are labeled hyperactive or hyperkinetic. In both, attention span may be short and ability to concentrate limited.

Fatigue is also characteristic of both, I believe, even though on the surface it may not seem to be. I have known many a hypothyroid child who, in an effort to fight the fatigue resulting from low thyroid function, had to keep in constant motion. Hyperkinetic children now are commonly treated with central nervous system stimulants—amphetamines or similar-acting drugs. And it has always been something of a puzzle why these drugs, which stimulate adults, seem to do exactly the opposite in hyperkinetic youngsters, calming and quieting them. The stimulation may well serve to overcome some of the hyperkinetic child's basic fatigue and, in so doing, relieve the need for overactivity as a fatigue-fighting measure.

The use of a stimulant drug may be one way of attacking the problem of hyperactivity. (And it is worth noting here that some physicians have recently found that a hyperactive child often may respond as well to coffee as to a stimulant drug—for coffee, too, of course, has a stimulating, fatigue-fighting effect.)

Another way to attack the problem when it turns out that a hyperactive child is hypothyroid is to treat the hypothyroidism, getting at the basic cause rather than just trying to control the manifestations.

The Bright and Failing

From 1938 to 1941, I had the privilege of having referred to me all failing students at Armour Tech, now the Illinois Institute of Technology, in Chicago. Tech standards of admission were very high; only men in the upper 10 percent of their high school graduating classes had any chance for admission. Yet, among these very bright young men, there were failures, sometimes within a year of entrance, sometimes later.

All of them were examined thoroughly. Rarely was there any glaring physical illness. Commonly, however, low thyroid function could be found. This was a time when basal metabolism tests were routine for thyroid function and work was just beginning on basal temperature. Some of the men, if they could relax during the basal metabolism test, were found by this means to be hypothyroid. Many others who could not relax and appeared from results of the test to have normal thyroid function were subsequently found to have subnormal basal temperatures. And when hypothyroidism was detected either way and then treated, the results were often striking.

One student who comes to mind stood at the top of his class in high school and did well at the beginning at Tech. But he was extremely ambitious, worked very hard, and fatigue became his Waterloo. Although he would know his subject thoroughly before an examination, he would be so tired upon taking the exam that he couldn't concentrate. As his marks plummeted, he tried all the harder, only to begin to fail almost completely. He became increasingly frustrated and at one point attempted suicide. Fortunately, the attempt was thwarted.

He had a low thyroid condition and his response to thyroid therapy was gratifying. He took his rightful place in his class, graduated with honors, and later became an outstanding success in engineering.

Another of this group of students was a big, husky six-footer and a thoroughly likeable fellow. Because of financial difficulties he had had to work for two years before starting at Tech and was older than his classmates. At Tech, he participated in a program in which he spent three months on campus, then three in industry, and by thus alternating could earn his way through.

During his junior year, despite his best efforts, he

began to fall behind in his class work. On the verge of failure, he sought help from a clinical psychologist who referred him to me for examination. When I saw him, he was on the ragged edge and broke down and cried like a baby about being a failure.

He was hypothyroid and responded to thyroid therapy. Within a month, his school work began to improve. Six months later, he was doing superior work in school and also on the job and his employer advised him that, if he wished to take it, there would be a management job waiting for him when he graduated.

This group of students taught me much about mental and behavioral performance and thyroid deficiency, especially that thyroid deficiency may be present for many years in a latent state and may become manifest and affect performance at some point when there is undue stress.

At Any Age

The change from latent to manifest can occur at any age at which sufficient stress is experienced. It accounts, I believe, for many of the emotional upsets and alleged psychosomatic complaints seen in young mothers, for example. A household to manage, finances to worry about, diapers to change, sleep often broken by need to care for children—all of this is stressful. When depressed feelings then emerge and when physical symptoms as well appear—headaches, intestinal difficulties, or others—a search for low thyroid function and, if found, its treatment can be much more rewarding than applying a psychosomatic label and perhaps throwing in some "mind pills."

Several years ago, Dr. Martha Schon of the Neuropsychiatric Service at Memorial Hospital in New York City carried out a study in which she found that patients with untreated thyroid deficiency could easily be mistaken for neurotics.

She investigated two dozen such patients. They were fatigued, irritable, and nervous. They were also emotionally explosive and showed oppositional tendencies. They regretted their behavior but were unable to control it. Sexual function was decreased. There were varied physical symptoms including vision disturbances, speech difficulties, and diffuse muscular pain.

Interestingly, Dr. Schon found that while neurotics, real neurotics, usually blame those around them or circumstances for their difficulties, hypothyroid patients with seeming neurotic problems assume responsibility for their emotional reactions.

Once the thyroid deficiency was corrected, Dr. Schon reported, most of the symptoms, emotional as well as physical, decreased or disappeared entirely to be replaced by a sense of well-being and a feeling of integration of personality.

Evidently, Dr. Schon suggested, thyroid hormones have the ability to balance emotions and can aid in the treatment of mental disorders. And, she also noted, it appeared that hypothyroidism not caused by surgical removal of the thyroid gland might well be brought on by mental pressures with which an individual is unable to cope.

Recently, too, a team of investigators headed by Dr.

Arthur J. Prange, Jr., director of research development in the department of psychiatry at the University of North Carolina School of Medicine, reported a striking finding. One form of mental depression, called the retarded, slows a patient down in actions and thoughts and leads to apathy. Antidepressant drugs are often used in such cases and may be helpful. The North Carolina physicians found that when, along with an antidepressant drug such as imipramine, they used tiny amounts of thyroid hormone in treatment, there was a marked difference in results. In contrast to patients receiving imipramine alone, some of whom failed to benefit even after several weeks of treatment, no patient receiving thyroid hormone with imipramine failed to benefit. And in some cases, within just the first eight hours, patients receiving the combined treatment showed remarkable improvement.

Subsequently, Dr. Prange and his colleagues were able to show that in nonretarded depression as well, thyroid hormone reduced by about half the time needed to produce remission.

Also at the University of North Carolina, Dr. P.C. Whybrow and other investigators studied a group of patients with mental disturbances who proved to be hypothyroid. Virtually all complained of poor recent memory and difficulty in concentration. They had difficulty on testing with simple dollars-and-cents arithmetic. Several of the women complained they could no longer remember long-used cooking recipes and had to constantly refer now to a recipe book, and one had come to rely on her children to remember where she placed things around the house.

One woman considered herself a burden to her family and had frequent thoughts of suicide. She had become preoccupied with memories of her son who had been killed in an automobile accident some years before. She wished she had been the one killed. She dreamed of digging him from his grave with her bare hands and heard his voice calling her during the day.

Another woman had experienced increasing insomnia. When she did sleep, she had vivid morbid dreams, the content of which she at times believed with almost delusional intensity. She dreamed of her only son's death and of mutilation of other family members. She was increasingly concerned that she was losing her mind.

These were all severely afflicted patients. They might easily have been considered victims of serious psychiatric illness. Their physicians were psychiatrists—but alert, investigative psychiatrists, aware of the possible mental repercussions of hypothyroidism. And they used thyroid therapy to correct the hypothyroidism and relieve the seeming psychiatric illnesses.

Are there undiagnosed cases of hypothyroidism in mental institutions? One hopes not, but possibly there might be. In 1949, a study in Britain indicated that such cases were frequent there and that many, once their thyroid deficiency was recognized and treated, could go home.

A Confusion of Symptoms

Certainly, low thyroid function is not the reason for every difficult-to-diagnose mental and mental/physical problem. But its ability to produce a wide variety of symptoms should be remembered.

Some years ago, a review of 109 cases of hypothyroidism seen at Georgetown University showed that inability to concentrate was prominent in 31 percent of the patients, forgetfulness in 26 percent, deafness in 17 percent, noises in the ears in 8 percent, and poor muscular coordination in another 8 percent. Moreover paresthesias— sensations of prickling, tingling, or creeping on the skin —were present in 79 percent, and more than 20 percent of the patients had convulsive seizures.

At the Mayo Clinic, a team of neurologists led by Dr. G.M. Cremer studied twenty-four patients—five men and nineteen women—who had been referred for neurological investigation because of varied puzzling symptoms and who turned out to be hypothyroid. The symptoms included mental slowing, poor equilibrium, incoordination of the limbs, muscle disturbances, hearing disturbances, and paresthesias. The symptoms responded to thyroid therapy.

One of the patients, for example, was a woman who had been referred for investigation of a possible brain tumor. She had long experienced bouts of dizziness and more recently, for eighteen months, had felt lightheaded and had noticed increasing loss of hearing in both ears. Careful study also revealed definite muscle disturbances and mental slowing. Within two weeks after start of thyroid therapy, she could walk without feeling dizzy. At the end of six months, there was still further improvement, including return of normal hearing. At eighteen months, with continued treatment, she was completely well.

Never Too Late

A failure to recognize hypothyroidism early, as soon as it begins to manifest itself, can lead to needless suffering. The suffering may go on for years and even much of a lifetime, yet it is never too late for treatment.

I recall well one patient, not my own, reported by another physician: a mother of two who, it was obvious in retrospect, had been a victim of hypothyroidism for virtually all of her adult life. When the children were young, she had begun to manifest disturbed behavior. The disturbance at first was mild, a little intolerance, impatience, irritability now and again. But over the years she had become extremely difficult to live with. She became chronically intolerant of husband, children, and home. She became selfish, deceitful, extravagant. Against her daughter's will, she pushed her into an unfavorable marriage. Her son left home because of her everlasting nagging and bickering. Finally, her husband could stand it no longer and walked out. She was sixty-nine years old before it was finally recognized that she was hypothyroid. With treatment for the deficiency, the change was dramatic. Her whole personality was altered. At that late stage in her life, she became a practical nurse and spent the rest of her years taking care of people.

I have seen many patients with psychological and other disturbances caused by low thyroid function that went undetected for years. Some had presented indications of thyroid deficiency at early age which had not been recognized as such.

One such patient was a forty-year-old woman I saw recently. She had been a fat child until the age of three when she had a serious illness with aggravated diarrhea; after that she was always skinny. At the age of eight, she had scarlet fever, followed shortly by kidney trouble. She had repeated pains in her knees and legs which were called "growing pains."

In high school, it was apparent that she was not maturing normally. Her menstrual periods did not start until her senior year when she was seventeen and then were scant and painful, requiring bed rest for one or two days. She entered a convent after graduating from high school. There, she was sickly, suffered from repeated nosebleeds, and very loose bowel movements.

When she was twenty, she began to do some teaching and the stress of that led to repeated severe intestinal upsets and repeated X-ray studies of the intestinal tract which produced no definitive findings. For a time, while her teaching load was very much lightened, she seemed to improve a bit. At age twenty-three, when she was given a job of some responsibility, her intestinal upsets returned and she became extremely tense. Her bowel problems had led to hemorrhoids and she required surgery, after which she was placed on tranquilizers.

At age thirty, she collapsed, thoroughly exhausted, unable to go on, and spent a month in a psychiatric ward where, somewhat rested, she seemed to improve. There followed weekly psychotherapy sessions. Rather than return to teaching, she decided to become a counselor, received training in counseling, and subsequently left the convent and obtained employment as a counselor at a state college. For a time, she enjoyed the work.

But when I saw her at age forty, she was an exhausted and thoroughly depressed woman. She weighed only 95 pounds although she was of average height. Her breasts and uterus were underdeveloped, her circulation was poor. Her basal temperature was 96.4. Undoubtedly, it had been low all her life and she had been a lifelong victim of low thyroid function. On thyroid therapy, she has gained energy, come out of her depression, is back at counseling with enthusiasm.

7

Infectious Diseases: Why, For Some, So Many

IF MUCH OR ALL of your life, you've been prone to get what has seemed to you to be more than a normal share of respiratory and other infections and those you get are generally severe and prolonged, you belong to a sizeable group of people. I've known many such patients and I have belonged in the group myself.

For a very long time, it has been evident that some people are unusually susceptible to infectious diseases and to succumbing to them while others are relatively resistant, acquiring them much less often and better able to fight off those they do pick up.

Several centuries ago, smallpox was a major threat. It was one of the most contagious of all diseases and epidemics affected vast numbers, yet many escaped. It was one of the most lethal of diseases, too, killing 25 percent of those who contracted it, yet some people, if not resistant to getting it, were more resistant than others to succumbing to it.

As smallpox gradually came under control through the use of vaccination, tuberculosis took over as Captain Death and retained the title until the advent of modern anti-TB therapy. In the United States as late as the 1930s, tuberculosis was the leading cause of death in people between the ages of fifteen and thirty-nine. Here again, was an infectious disease to which some were susceptible and some resistant.

In my own family, susceptibility was high. My mother died of tuberculosis when I was six. I lost two sisters to the same disease before they started school. I was born in Missouri but after my mother's death my father moved us to Colorado with the hope that we could get away from tuberculosis. I grew up on a cow ranch south of Denver and as a child did heavy work and was muscularly tough. But I was unusually susceptible to colds, sore throats, boils, and carbuncles. Even as a young man in graduate school, I had one respiratory infection after another, one attack of tonsillitis after another, which finally led to tonsillectomy.

In graduate school, as I've indicated earlier, I worked with baby rabbits whose thyroid glands were removed in order to demonstrate the important functions of the thyroid by noting what were the consequences of its loss. And not least among the many consequences were continuous sniffles, repeated acute infections, and death at an early age of pneumonia.

Yet it wasn't until five years after I had completed medical school that I realized why I might be so prone to infections. I was giving a series of lectures on endocrinology at Stevens College in Columbia, Missouri. The time was early October. The evenings seemed quite cool, even cold, to me and I wore a topcoat. I noticed, however, that other faculty members and the students seemed to have no need for topcoats and appeared perfectly comfortable without them.

I remembered then that a common complaint among hypothyroid patients in my practice was a tendency to feel cold even in what for others was a pleasantly warm room. Suddenly the thought struck and I told myself: "You fool, you're one of them."

I had begun to use basal temperature as a means of detecting low thyroid function. I took my own. It was low. Lifelong medication with thyroid began immediately thereafter, and I have had little further trouble from infections.

My wife comes from an infection-susceptible family. Her father, a physician, died of pneumonia at the age of thirty-seven. Her mother died at the age of twenty-six of tuberculosis. My wife developed tuberculosis after a history of repeated respiratory infections through much of her childhood and young adulthood. The tuberculosis appeared shortly after the birth of our second son and she was treated in a sanatorium. I wasn't smart enough to check her thyroid function and place her on needed thyroid therapy until after she was released from the sanatorium. She is very much alive and well today, at more than double the age at which her mother died of tuberculosis. Her only problem is an occasional attack of sinusitis. Thyroid therapy has not eliminated such attacks for her but they are much milder than they used to be, occur much less frequently, and she recovers from them much more quickly.

Our oldest son, during his first year of school, was out almost one-fouth of the time with colds and other respiratory infections. His basal temperature was low. I hadn't ever before used thyroid therapy for a child with low resistance to infection. Within two months, his resistance was up and thereafter he had at most two colds a year and more often just one or none.

Since then, in any patient at any age with proneness to infection, I have made it a point to check thyroid function and use thyroid therapy when function was low, regardless of whether or not any other symptoms of low thyroid function were present. My youngest patient was a three-week-old infant who from birth had been unable to breathe through his nose because of a continuous upper respiratory infection. He was low in thyroid function as were both his parents. His resistance became normal within a few weeks on thyroid treatment.

The Thyroid and Resistance

It takes more than infectious agents to produce infection.

Infectious agents are always about us and even on and within us. They are present on the skin, in the nose and mouth, in the gastrointestinal tract. We are constantly exposed to our own bacteria, viruses, and other agents capable of causing illness and we are intermittently exposed to those of other people. But as long as our resistance is high, we don't provide the conditions under

which infectious agents can multiply to the point of producing illness.

We have, in fact, several lines of defense or resistance.
The first line prevents organisms from gaining entrance.
The skin is part of the defense and unless broken by a
wound is practically microbe-proof. Organisms lie harm-
lessly on it.

Body openings, too, are defended. Mucous membranes are protective. In the breathing passages, their
secretions of mucus form a sticky coating that catches
many organisms before they can penetrate further. Tiny
filters, including hair in the nose, help keep out microbes.

Body fluids have defense functions. Not only do tears
wash organisms out of the eyes but they also are slightly
antiseptic and discourage organism growth. Stomach
acid is lethal to many organisms that enter with food.

A second line of defense is normally ready when organisms penetrate through the first line. Leukocytes, or
white cells, present in the blood, attack organisms at the
site of invasion. And if this is not enough, the body
produces other defense agents, antibodies, which can
lock onto and inactivate or even dissolve the invading
organisms.

The natural resistance we have, or should have, is
remarkably effective. But if resistance is lowered, disease
agents, always present and ready to strike, can over-
whelm us.

Many influences can lower resistance. Inadequate
sleep, poor nutrition, and undue stress are among them.
Low thyroid function is a major factor. With reduced
output of thyroid hormones, every cell and every system
of the body, including the defense system may be af-

fected. If thyroid function is low enough, this in itself can be enough to open the door to repeated bacterial and viral invasions. And mild degrees of hypothyroidism can set the stage so that brief loss of adequate sleep or a brief period of undue stress may do what it would not otherwise be capable of doing in anyone with normal thyroid function: add just enough to the lowering of resistance to permit infection. Mild hypothyroidism may also set the stage so that exposure to another person with an infectious disease may lead to infection that would not "take" in a person with normal thyroid function who is similarly exposed.

I have seen this demonstrated repeatedly in laboratory animals and in human patients of all ages. Not only rabbits but also rats with low thyroid function are all unusually susceptible to infectious diseases. When given thyroid medication, however, their resistance is raised. Quite recently, in experiments with swine, I have found exactly the same thing to be true.

The evidence in children is particularly dramatic. Youngsters who were victims of repeated colds and other respiratory infections before their hypothyroidism was detected and treated, who once lost much time from school because of illness, have become healthier and far less subject to infections, even though exposed as much as before in school to other youngsters with infections.

Adult city dwellers often remark that by the very nature of city living—the crowds in public places, the congestion on mass transit facilities—it is impossible to avoid repeated colds, attacks of flu, and other "bugs that keep going around." Certainly, there may be greater exposure to sources of infection in urban than in rural areas. Yet urban adults, as well as rural adults, who are hypothyroid and have had excessive difficulty with infectious diseases almost invariably have far less difficulty once their low thyroid function is compensated for by thyroid therapy.

My first medical report on the thyroid and infection was made in 1953 after I had followed for some time a group of 150 patients who had been susceptible to respiratory infections and had received thyroid therapy for low thyroid function. They not only felt more vigorous and in better general health but they experienced far fewer infections.

Since then, I have seen the same gratifying results in many hundreds of others. For some, the primary complaint that brought them to treatment was repeated infection; for others, proneness to infection was one of a number of symptoms of hypothyroidism. No matter. Once the hypothyroidism was corrected, there was increased resistance to infectious disease.

For one ranching family, repeated respiratory infection was the primary complaint for both parents and all three children. The youngsters, all of school age, almost always were exchanging colds among themselves and handing them on to parents. And the colds in the family were severe, more often than not producing complications such as sinusitis and middle ear infection and, on several occasions, pneumonia. The family's history showed that as often as once every four to six weeks, some member or other would require antibiotic therapy for complications. Every one of the family members had a basal temperature indicative of low thyroid function. Since all have been placed on suitable dosages of thyroid, the children get only one or two colds a year, the parents rarely that many, and complications have virtually vanished.

Recently, I saw a woman of sixty-six who had been an unrecognized hypothyroid for many years and who came from a family in which, I am certain, hypothyroidism was rife. Infectious disease was an almost constant problem in the family, and a tragic one. One of her brothers had died at the age of seven of bronchial trouble; another had died at thirteen of rheumatic fever; a third at age fifteen of pneumonia. She had managed to survive repeated infections, including an attack of rheumatic fever in 1933 which had required long hospitalization. The rheumatic fever recurred in 1956 and was followed later by two bouts of pneumonia.

When I saw her, she was in the early stages of emphysema and quite probably the destructive lung disease was the result, in no small part, of the repeated infectious insults. Treatment for her hypothyroidism is helping her to be more resistant to infections and, in so doing, although it cannot reverse the already-present destructive changes of emphysema, may very well help prevent further inroads of the disease.

Rheumatic Fever

Prior to the advent of antibiotics, rheumatic fever was the most common cause of heart disease. The late Dr. Paul Dudley White, distinguished heart specialist, noted in a book on heart disease which he wrote in 1931 that in New England rheumatic fever was responsible for 40 percent of all cases of heart disease, with 93 percent of them occurring before the age of twenty.

Rheumatic fever usually follows a streptococcal infection such as strep sore throat or scarlet fever. Among the early signs, usually beginning ten to fourteen days after the strep infection, are fever, pallor, irritability, moderate weight loss. Thereafter, more specific symptoms appear—pain in the joints which are tender to the touch and hurt when moved. The joints may become red and swollen but are never crippled. Although the acute phase of the disease passes, some subtle injury may be left on one or more of the valves of the heart.

A first attack of rheumatic fever is not likely to severely damage the heart valves. Serious damage that impairs the functioning of the valves and interferes with proper blood flow comes with repeat attacks.

Antibiotics have reduced the incidence of rheumatic fever and rheumatic heart disease but have not eliminated either. It is common practice to maintain rheumatic fever patients on antibiotics indefinitely after the acute phase of the disease has passed and this has helped prevent potentially dangerous recurrences.

It is impractical to give antibiotics to every child in order to prevent a first attack. But personal observation suggests that if children susceptible to repeated infections are treated with thyroid for their low thyroid function, rheumatic fever can be avoided. In more than thirty years of practice, not a single case of rheumatic fever has occurred in any child receiving thyroid.

Moreover, in my experience, thyroid therapy has been effective in preventing recurrences in children with a previous history of rheumatic fever. After about a month, antibiotics could be discontinued, saving that expense and avoiding the risk of possible complications of extended use of antibiotics, and no child has had a recurrence.

It seems to me more physiological to correct a deficiency with a natural and harmless product such as thyroid than to keep a child for many years on therapy with a much more expensive and not invariably harmless drug.

Ear and Other Infections

In 1965, at an American Medical Association meeting in New York City, I was able to present a scientific exhibit showing the results of thyroid therapy in a large group of patients. Rheumatic fever had not developed in any child taking thyroid even though Colorado was acknowledged to be one of the worst places for the disorder. Resistance had increased in children who had had rheumatic fever before and no recurrences had been seen after the institution of thyroid therapy. Children who had missed school repeatedly because of upper respiratory infections had improved and had only one or two colds a year. Ear infections were seldom seen. Pneumonias were extremely rare. In all age groups, resistance was increased against influenza and pneumonia. It appeared that vaccines against influenza in the aged were unnecessary once their thyroid function had been returned to normal.

I think particularly of one patient, a woman now forty-four, who had been prone to infections all of her life. At age six, she contracted pneumonia. When I first saw her ten years ago, she had a history of thirteen other bouts of pneumonia. She also had other stigma of thyroid deficiency, including excessive fatigue and menstrual difficulties. In the ten years she has been on thyroid therapy, she has had no severe respiratory infections at all, very rarely even a mild cold.

Repeated otitis media, or middle-ear infection, can be a signal that a patient may be hypothyroid. Such infection can occur when host resistance is lowered to the point that organisms can ascend from the throat through the eustachian tube which runs from the throat to the middle ear. Otitis media is often thought of as a disease only of children yet autopsies in the goiter region of Graz, Austria, leave no doubt that hypothyroid adults also are vulnerable. In 1939, before the advent of antibiotics, 6.75 percent of autopsies at Graz revealed that the basic cause of death was middle-ear infection, with bacteria penetrating beyond the ear to reach the brain and produce meningitis. Most deaths occurred in children but all age groups were affected.

Even in 1960, fifteen years after the introduction of antibiotics, otitis media was far from conquered in Graz with its large hypothyroid population. In that year, it accounted for 4 percent of all deaths—for even antibiotics may not be adequate when resistance is markedly lowered by thyroid deficiency.

Many American Indians are susceptible to ear infections. During World War II, when I was stationed at an army camp in Kingman, Arizona, housing was at a premium and we lived on an Indian reservation 25 miles away. Because there was no physician at the one Indian hospital, I offered to cover emergencies at night when I would be at home and available. I became acquainted with Indians and their health problems then and for four years after the war when I practiced in Kingman and had many Indian patients. Their incidence of infections was high; otitis media was a common problem; and the incidence of thyroid deficiency also was high, not surprising since many Indian tribes had low iodine intake for centuries and intermarriage accentuated thyroid deficiencies.

Bladder infections are much less common than respiratory infections but they too may suggest hypothyroidism—again because of lowered resistance. Among the susceptible, recurrences are frequent and the end result of repeated infection may be kidney failure. In my experience, resistance to bladder and kidney disease in patients with low thyroid function can be increased greatly and readily with thyroid therapy.

The last patient in my practice who succumbed to kidney failure died more than twenty-five years ago. Severe kidney damage had occurred before she was seen. Since then, no patient on thyroid therapy has experienced repeated bladder or other urinary infections or suffered from deterioration of kidney function.

Osteomyelitis—bone infection—was once a nightmare dreaded by physicians treating fractures with exposed bones. The antibiotics have been of great help but there are still cases of prolonged morbidity. Almost invariably in those I have seen, low thyroid function has been present and thyroid therapy has been beneficial.

One young patient, a boy who broke his foot in a bicycle accident, developed osteomyelitis which would seem to yield for a time to antibiotics but kept recurring. Not until he was found to be hypothyroid and was placed on thyroid therapy did the infection really subside and healing take place.

A college boy who had a serious automobile accident in which several bones were fractured, developed osteomyelitis in a leg bone. Again, despite antibiotics, the infection kept recurring. His parents were hypothyroid and on thyroid therapy. The boy, too, was hypothyroid, and I had placed him on thyroid therapy some years before. But, on his own, he had decided that he need not take thyroid and had stopped it about a year before the accident. The recurrent osteomyelitis brought him to his senses and he returned to thyroid therapy; not long afterward, the osteomyelitis was gone.

Another patient, a woman now forty-four years old, had developed osteomyelitis at the age of two and from then until she was twenty-nine years old she had required repeated scraping and draining of all of the eight long bones of her body. She had eight- to ten-inch-long operative scars where it had been necessary to go in surgically, expose bones, remove a badly diseased piece, and drain. She had had thirty operations between the age of two and twenty-nine. Her osteomyelitis was not the result of any accidental fracture. Instead, her resistance had been so low that organisms apparently coming from her frequent respiratory infections found their way, through her bloodstream, to take up housekeeping in her long bones. Since her hypothyroidism was recognized and therapy for it started, she has not had a recurrence in fifteen years.

I referred earlier but not fully to the case of a seventy-nine-year-old man who had suffered for so much of his life from a draining left ear and from a sinus draining pus from his left mid-thigh that he thought those conditions were hopeless. He consulted me not because of them but rather because he had been hospitalized recently for dizziness and weakness, and nothing could be found during the hospitalization to explain the symptoms. His basal temperature was low—95 degrees. With thyroid therapy, his dizziness disappeared as did his weakness and, miraculously, he thought, both his infections, one of them present since age eighteen, cleared up.

To make the story complete, he felt so well that nine years later he neglected his thyroid and his ear began draining again. With resumption of thyroid therapy, the ear condition cleared up once more. He died at the age of eighty-nine when his heart finally wore out, but his last ten years were happy ones thanks to the better resistance, freedom from infection, and increased vigor that thyroid therapy had provided.

When low thyroid function is responsible for lowered resistance to infectious disease, about two months of treatment are usually needed to raise the resistance. The effect will wear off in six months to a year if thyroid therapy is stopped.

The most common infections today are those produced by viruses, notably the common cold and influenza. All of our modern knowledge has not solved the problem of the common cold and even influenza vaccines are of questionable efficacy. Here, no less than for other infections, the resistance of the individual is a cardinal factor. The correction of thyroid deficiency can do much to raise resistance to colds and flu as it does to pneumonia and other bacterial infections—and if increased resistance cannot entirely guarantee freedom from the twin nuisances of colds and flu, it can do much to reduce the frequency with which they strike and their severity and duration.

Similarly, correction of thyroid deficiency can do much to increase resistance to skin infections and may help in chronic skin problems, as we shall see in the next chapter.

8

The Thyroid
and the Skin

THE PATIENTS WERE COLLEGE STUDENTS between the ages
of seventeen and twenty-five. They were well-nourished
and otherwise healthy but they suffered from furunculosis—boils.

There is a widespread belief that boils are the result of
"bad blood" although there is no scientific support for
that view. Lack of cleanliness has also been suggested as a
factor.

But these students at the University of Denver weren't
unclean and no blood test suggested "bad blood" or anything at all wrong with blood quality. There were no
obvious local skin conditions contributing to the development of the angry, swollen, inflamed lesions. The
students shared only one thing in common: subnormal
basal temperature.

The boils were duly treated with heat; they were incised for pus drainage; and they responded to treatment. The students then were divided into two groups for comparison purposes. One group received thyroid therapy; the other did not.

In those who did not receive thyroid therapy, boils recurred over a three-month period. Heat treatment was used; in each case, the boil went on to enlarge and to require incision. In one case, a grain a day of thyroid was started and heat applications were stopped. There were two boils under one arm, one under the other. Within ten days, the boils disappeared completely.

In the other group of students receiving thyroid therapy from the start, there was not a single case of boil recurrence. Almost a year later, however, one of the students stopped thyroid medication; within two months he had a recurrence.

For good reasons, as we shall soon see, low thyroid function can play an important role not only in the development and recurrence of boils and carbuncles but in other skin conditions as well—in acne, eczema, dry skin, "winter itch," ichthyosis or "fish skin," and still others.

The Thyroid and Skin Defenses

The circulation of blood through the skin can be measured accurately by means of electronic equipment. And such measurements have established that when thyroid function is low, circulation is reduced. In advanced cases of hypothyroidism, the skin, in fact, may receive as little as one-fourth to one-fifth the normal blood supply.

With reduced circulation, the nourishment supplied by blood is reduced and, at the same time, waste products are not removed promptly and completely since blood is the remover. The result is a skin which is not normally healthy and normally resistant to would-be invaders.

The skin always has on it many types of bacteria, some of them incapable of producing disease but others very much able to do so if they can invade and multiply. When resistance is lowered, the gates, in effect, are lowered.

Boils are one result of invasion. Bacteria, usually staphlococci, move in and set up housekeeping at the bottom of a hair follicle or a sebaceous gland. A red, elevated, tender pustule begins to develop and grows in size until at some point the surface of the pustule breaks down and the core of the boil with all the accumulated pus is extruded. If two or more boils happen to coalesce, a much larger carbuncle—hard, pus-filled, and painful —develops. It involves deeper skin layers and has multiple draining sinuses to the surface.

Boils and carbuncles can be treated with antibiotics and, when necessary, with incision and drainage. But recurrences can be expected in many cases unless the cause is eradicated. When basal temperature is low in a victim of boils or carbuncles, correction of the low thyroid condition, as I have noted repeatedly, can produce dramatic results.

One of the worst cases of boils I have ever seen was a soldier I encountered during military duty in World War II. The man had suffered for years, almost never free of a crop despite repeated medical efforts to help him. Among the measures that had been used was autoimmunization with a vaccine prepared from his own boils with the hope that it might stimulate him to develop greater resistance to the specific organisms involved. He finally did develop resistance when his hypothyroid condition was recognized and treated.

Impetigo

This superficial skin disease, which can be caused either by streptococcal or staphylococcal bacteria, produces pustules a little less than half an inch in diameter or large pus-filled blisters that rupture and crust. The pustules or blisters may be confined to one area of the skin but often, particularly in infants, they spread to involve the entire face and body, and if proper treatment is not instituted, there is risk of fatal systemic infection. In adults, there is less likelihood of spread, but if the impetigo is neglected, ulcers or boils may develop.

Impetigo usually responds to antibiotics applied to the skin. But hypothyroidism is to be suspected in children and adults who develop impetigo, and correction of low thyroid function can prevent recurrences.

Cellulitis

This spreading inflammation also may indicate low thyroid function. Caused by infection with streptococci, staphylococci, or other organisms, cellulitis affects the skin and tissues beneath the skin and produces redness, swelling, and pain. Fever, chills, malaise, and headache also may be present. Severe cellulitis can be dangerous. Abscess formation and destruction of tissue may occur. Cellulitis of the scalp may produce brain complications by spread through veins. Cellulitis of the floor of the mouth is a serious condition that may require surgery although it usually responds to antibiotics as does cellulitis elsewhere.

Erysipelas

This is an acute streptococcal infection of the skin characterized by hot red patches with accompanying fever and malaise. Before the advent of sulfa drugs and antibiotics, death from erysipelas was not unusual, for among the complications were the spread of bacteria or their poisons in the blood (septicemia), pneumonia, rheumatic fever, and kidney inflammation. I have seen only a limited number of patients with erysipelas but in every case hypothyroidism was present.

Acne

One of the most common skin diseases usually associated with some degree of thyroid deficiency—although that association is too rarely recognized—is acne vulgaris.

If a hair follicle opening on the surface of the skin is small or becomes clogged by dirt or cosmetics, fatty material produced by the sebaceous gland accumulates and a bump appears under the skin or a whitehead or black-head shows on the skin surface. The dark color of black-heads is the result not of dirt but of the discoloring effect of air on the material in the clogged follicle. When infection sets in, a pimple results. In severe cases, cysts may form and leave ugly scars.

There have been innumerable efforts to find effective measures against acne. At one time or other, various foods have been indicated as possible acne fomenters and have been banned. Scrupulous cleanliness has been advocated and to achieve that not only plain soap but antibacterial soaps and other cleansers have been used.

At the time I was associated with the Health Service of the University of Denver, I saw many students with acne. About that time, Dr. R.L. Sutton, Jr., a well-known Kansas City dermatologist, published a medical report telling of good results in the treatment of acne with use of three measures: thyroid therapy, dietary changes, and local treatment. When I saw his report, I wondered which of the three measures might be the most effective. Could it be the thyroid regimen? Dietary changes and local treatment had been tried many times before without any remarkable effect.

I worked with a group of students with acne, foregoing local treatment and dietary changes. The only measure used was thyroid therapy. The results with thyroid therapy alone matched those obtained by Dr. Sutton with the three-measure regimen. The majority of students showed marked improvement; a few did not.

Ever since, in every case of acne, I have checked for thyroid function and where it has been low as indicated by basal temperature I have prescribed thyroid. Better than 90 percent of patients have benefited to some degree, and often to a marked degree.

And this has been true not only for acne in the younger years but for acne persisting into the later years. There have been gratifying responses in men and women in their thirties, forties, and even later who had suffered on and off or even continuously with acne.

One of my oldest patients with the problem was a sixty-one-year-old man first seen because he suspected he might have had a mild heart attack. An electrocardiogram did, indeed, show that there had been a mild episode. When he removed his shirt for the electrocardiogram, I noted that his back was covered with acne lesions. He had had the problem, he told me, ever since his teens and nothing had ever been found to help.

Although we quickly determined that he was hypothyroid, he had to be started on thyroid therapy cautiously because of the very recent heart attack. No thyroid was administered at all until a month had elapsed and then the dose was minimal—half a grain a day. Gradually, we could increase it to what was needed, two grains a day. Within a few months his acne had cleared entirely and has not returned.

The Thyroid and Skin Changes

Reduced circulation of blood through the skin is one effect of low thyroid function. Another is of great importance.

It was a century ago that Sir William Gull presented five cases to the Clinical Society of London of what he called a "cretinoid state supervening in adult life in women." The outstanding characteristic of these patients was a masklike appearance of the face, with swelling under the skin and around the eyes.

Five years later, another leading London physician, Dr. W.M. Ord, reported five similar patients, one of whom he had been observing for fifteen years. The patient was a fifty-four-year-old widow with two children. There had been no unusual illnesses in her family. Hers started subtly. At first she simply noticed that she tended to get unusually cold and to shiver while working. Then, on several occasions, she noticed blood in her urine. Subsequently, her right arm had become somewhat lame, making her work as a seamstress difficult. She also described herself as feeling "weak-headed" because of difficulty in remembering things and keeping her mind clear.

As her illness progressed, she lost muscular power, suffered from a constant backache, and the skin of her entire body became swollen and her face lost all expression. She died in coma at the age of fifty-eight.

When Ord performed an autopsy, he found that, although her skin was markedly swollen, water did not escape from a cut surface as it does when there is water-logging from kidney failure. Chemical analysis revealed the presence of an excess of a jellylike material, called mucin, which has a high affinity for water and, by attracting and holding water, had led to swelling all over the body including the skin.

Ord also found that the thyroid gland was almost completely destroyed, suggesting that the condition was due to thyroid failure. He called the condition "myx-edema," "myx" being from the Greek for mucin.

Not long afterward, Dr. Victor Horsley, a British physiologist, carried out experiments in which he removed the thyroid glands from animals. Within a few weeks after loss of the thyroid, an increase in mucin could be found, and the swelling from waterlogging and the other symptoms of myxedema appeared. Little did the investigators then realize that a century later this compound, mucin, would become the subject of intense study in relation to many diseases such as heart attacks, diabetes, arthritis, and others, including those of the skin.

Mucin has been found to consist of several compounds now called mucopolysaccharides. The level of these compounds has been found to be increased in most tissues during many diseases and the possible full significance of the increase is being explored.

Evidence continues to accumulate that the mucopolysaccharide level is closely related to the level of thyroid function. In 1950, a Danish investigator, Asboe-Hansen of Copenhagen, demonstrated a high level of the compounds in the skin of hypothyroid patients and a reduction almost immediately after the start of thyroid therapy.

Five years later, another Danish researcher, H. Anderson, reported that the mucopolysaccharides in the skin accurately reflect the activity of the thyroid gland. He studied ninety-nine children, aged three months to fifteen years, who were being maintained with thyroid since they were born with a lack of adequate quantities. The mucopolysaccharides in their skins were at a normal level. Then, without any other changes, the thyroid medication was discontinued temporarily and within six weeks some of the children showed an excess of mucopolysaccharides in their skins.

Thus, two abnormalities in the skin—reduced blood circulation and excessive mucopolysaccharides—may be at work in hypothyroid patients and may account, in part or in whole, for the development of many skin problems or for their failure to yield completely to conventional treatment.

Effective Thyroid Therapy in Skin Problems

As early as 1893, soon after thyroid medication became available for use, an English physician, Dr. B. Bramwell, began to apply it for skin problems. He was able to report some spectacular results. So did several other investigators abroad. But attempts by American physicians to confirm Bramwell's work were negative. Going back now over their reports, it is obvious that the thyroid preparations available at the time in the United States often were not physiologically active. They were not standardized as to strength. None of the other beneficial effects, such as increased energy and reduced fatigability, now expected with modern thyroid preparations, appeared. Under those circumstances, no improvement in the skin could be expected.

These early fruitless attempts did much to discourage research on the influence of low thyroid function in dermatology. So did the difficulty in precise diagnosis of low thyroid function because of the unreliability of standard tests for hypothyroidism.

The use of the basal temperature test has made recognition of hypothyroidism as a possible cause of skin disorders easier. In the 1956 edition of his book *Diseases of the Skin,* Dr. Sutton pointed out that through its use he had found hypothyroidism present in many patients with skin diseases and that thyroid therapy had benefited the skin diseases while also bringing improvement in energy levels, menstrual difficulties, and other symptoms associated with thyroid deficiency.

Yet, today, low thyroid function still too often is going unsuspected in skin disorders of many types in which very often it is a major influence and its correction could bring striking improvement.

The Thyroid and "Winter Itch"

A frequent complaint during winter months is a generalized itching over the extremities, especially the lower parts of the arms and legs. There is no characteristic rash or other lesion. Yet, the itching, especially at night in bed, may be so intense that it interferes with sleep and leads to severe excoriations from scratching.

I was taught originally that this was "winter itch" and all that could be done for it was to use oil baths and ointments. And so I dutifully prescribed oil baths and ointments but with little success. Over the years, however, it became obvious to me that people with this affliction are hypothyroid and that virtually all of them respond to thyroid therapy.

Nor is it difficult to understand why the affliction should be most prevalent in winter. For in hypothyroid patients, blood circulation through the skin is less than normal at all times and is reduced even further in cold weather since at that time more blood is shifted away from the skin and to the interior of the body in order to preserve body heat.

I have seen many patients who have suffered from winter itch for years, some of them for much of their lifetimes, who have responded dramatically to thyroid therapy. I have seen patients who have had other stigma of hypothyroidism along with winter itch and yet the low thyroid function escaped diagnosis.

One recent patient, a twenty-eight-year-old mother of two, complained of severe itching along with prolonged menstrual flow and anemia. She had been hospitalized the previous winter because of the severity of the itching and her fatigability. There were extensive studies, including conventional thyroid function tests; all were negative. She was signed out of the hospital with a diagnosis of "fatigue of unknown origin and anemia from excessive menstruation."

Yet all of her complaints could indicate low thyroid function. Despite failure of conventional thyroid function tests to indicate hypothyroidism, the basal temperature test was used. When the basal temperature proved to be low, 94.4 degrees, she was started on one grain of thyroid daily. A month later, her temperature had reached 96.8 and the dosage was raised to two grains. In another month, although it was midwinter, her itching was gone, her energy level was increased, and her menstrual problem and anemia were markedly improved.

Relief for Eczema

Some of the most dramatic successes of thyroid therapy have been in eczema, which involves itching, swelling, blistering, oozing, and scaling of the skin.

In 1896, a British physician was one of the first to report the disappearance of eczema during thyroid administration in a sixty-five-year-old woman. In his report, the physician noted that if thyroid treatment was stopped, the eczema reappeared, but when thyroid therapy was resumed again, the eczema disappeared again.

In 1906, a German medical report pointed to thyroid medication as specific for eczema in infants. An American report in 1918 described a seemingly miraculous cure of generalized eczema in a three-year-old boy with use of thyroid. In the 1939 edition of his textbook on dermatology, Dr. Sutton, whom I've previously mentioned, pointed out that some infantile eczemas are due to thyroid deficiency and should be treated accordingly.

My personal experience covers fifty-seven patients with eczema who proved to be hypothyroid and for whom thyroid therapy was tried. Three failed to show any improvement but the rest did benefit and in most cases the benefit was marked.

A seven-month-old baby with very severe eczema, with crusts and bleeding points over much of his body, had to have his arms fixed snugly at his sides, day and night, to prevent him from scratching himself to the point of bleeding to death. He had been hospitalized twice. No treatment had provided relief. The child began to improve quickly on thyroid therapy; within five months all evidence of the disease was gone.

A nine-year-old youngster first seen seven years ago had chronic eczema in the bends of the elbows and behind his knees. He was a frail child, somewhat retarded in physical growth, and a victim of repeated asthma attacks that require hospitalization. The child's skin over abdomen and legs was scaly and rough, much like fish skin. His basal temperature was subnormal.

Thyroid therapy was started, as it happened in midsummer, and he began to show some improvement in his skin problems and even in his asthma, but such improvement is not unusual in summer. But improvement continued in fall and winter. His eczema was clearing and the scaliness and roughness gradually were disappearing. It was notable, too, that he had only one attack of asthma in the next year and that was a mild one. As he grew, the boy required an increase in thyroid dosage. His skin now was normal and his asthma was steadily improving and he was growing and developing like a normal child, playing with other children, and engaging in competitive sports.

"Fish Skin"

Known medically as ichthyosis, this can be a most distressing condition for its victims. The skin is dry and scaly; it may crack; it often itches; and it is unsightly.

Almost immediately after thyroid medication became available in the last century, it was tried successfully in patients with ichthyosis. A British textbook on diseases of the skin, written by Dr. H. Radcliffe Crocker in 1905, strongly recommended the use of thyroid for ichthyosis and, as well, for a number of other skin disorders, including lupus and psoriasis.

Dr. Crocker noted that thyroid therapy was beneficial

but the benefits were soon lost if treatment was discontinued. This may have been one reason why thyroid therapy was abandoned by subsequent dermatologists. They may have failed to realize that thyroid wasn't just a pill to clear up a skin condition, and that would be that, but rather that thyroid deficiency, leading to poor skin circulation and deposition of mucopolysaccharides, could be a basic cause of ichthyosis and other disorders, and the deficiency had to be made up continuously.

Unreliable thyroid function tests also helped to confuse the picture. When the tests failed to reveal mild and moderate degrees of thyroid deficiency, many physicians were led astray unwittingly. Rather than accept control of a disease by thyroid therapy as evidence that thyroid deficiency was present and a root cause, they accepted the results of faulty tests as gospel.

In every case of ichthyosis I have encountered, thyroid therapy has brought marked improvement. I remember well one patient, an eighteen-year-old WAC I saw while in military service during the Korean conflict. This otherwise attractive young lady had suffered all her life from ichthyosis of the legs. The skin of her legs looked like fish skin and felt to the touch like bristles. She responded beautifully to thyroid therapy. For the first time in her life she was able to wear nylon stockings.

Lupus

A serious disease called lupus erythematosus may involve only the skin, producing a butterfly-shaped, flushed area over the nose and cheeks, and, sometimes, firm, reddened lesions elsewhere, over the ears, scalp, and mucous membranes of the mouth. Or lupus may also involve many internal organs and joints.

It is one of the connective tissue diseases which include rheumatoid arthritis, progressive systemic sclerosis, polymyositis, amyloiditis, necrotizing arteritis, and rheumatic fever. All of these diseases are associated with deposition of mucopolysaccharides in the connective tissue. Considering the fact that thyroid deficiency leads to deposition of mucopolysaccharides in connective tissue and other tissue, it is not surprising, or shouldn't be, that thyroid therapy often can be beneficial.

Significantly, the "butterfly patch" on the skin characteristic of lupus was present in many of the original cases of myxedema investigated in England in the 1880s. It seems remarkable that the possible role of thyroid deficiency should have been overlooked so long, especially since as early as 1896 there was a report in the English medical literature of two cases of lupus apparently cured by thyroid therapy.

Throughout my medical career, I have routinely treated each case of lupus I have encountered with adequate thyroid therapy and each has responded satisfactorily without evidence of any involvement of the internal organs. Among the thousands of hypothyroid patients I have treated with thyroid in that time for other manifestations of thyroid deficiency, not one has developed lupus. To be sure, lupus is not a very common disease, and yet I have the feeling that thyroid therapy used where indicated to correct thyroid deficiency may act as a prophylactic agent against lupus.

Psoriasis

Psoriasis is another serious and often resistant disease of the skin. It is characterized by bright red patches covered with silvery scales which appear most often on the knees, elbows, and scalp. The chest, abdomen, backs of arms and legs, palms of the hands, and soles of the feet are other locations frequently affected. Psoriasis also may occur along with rheumatoid arthritis.

Here again, in psoriasis, the mucopolysaccharides are increased in the connective tissue. Early workers with thyroid therapy had reported about the turn of the century that some cases of psoriasis responded spectacularly while others were dismal failures.

My own experience with psoriasis has been limited to about a dozen cases, with no improvement at all from thyroid therapy in four but marked improvement in the others. In one case, the improvement was spectacular. This was the University of Denver retired dean whom I mentioned earlier. After half a century of being plagued by psoriasis, his skin cleared entirely with thyroid therapy.

The most serious psoriasis case in my series is a recent one. This is a twenty-four-year-old man whose psoriasis had started nine years before. Despite repeated treatment efforts, his condition had grown progressively worse and had reached the point where his entire skin was involved. When he undressed for physical examination, the floor was covered with scales.

Thyroid therapy was started and in about a month there was some improvement. But then no further progress was made. It became obvious that something else had to be done. At the end of the second month, prednisone was added in very small dosage to the thyroid medication. Prednisone is an anti-inflammatory compound related to hormones of the adrenal gland. With the addition of prednisone, further improvement occurred during the next month. A month later, the skin was almost clear for the first time in nine years. (More will be said about the combination of thyroid and prednisone therapy in the chapter on arthritis.)

Thyroid treatment is hardly a panacea for all skin diseases. Even when basal temperature is subnormal, indicating hypothyroidism and the need for thyroid therapy, such therapy will not invariably provide cures. Yet the chances for improvement are great enough to justify taking the basal temperature in any patient who has a chronic skin disorder and carrying out a trial of thyroid therapy if the basal temperature is low.

A common mistake during the early history of thyroid treatment for skin disorders was the expectation of immediate clearance. Many failures resulted from giving up thyroid treatment after just one or two weeks if no improvement was apparent. Conditions which have persisted for months and years take time for correction. At least six months should elapse before patient or physician can justifiably become discouraged. As long as the basal temperature does not go above the normal range for an extended period, no harm will result from continuous thyroid therapy.

9

Menstrual Disorders, Fertility Problems, and Avoiding Needless Surgery

WHEN A THIRTY-THREE-YEAR-OLD WOMAN presented herself for examination at a major clinic, she thought, understandably, that she was in serious trouble. Among her complaints were weakness, anemia, menstrual problems, and "heart trouble."

Four years before, six months after she had delivered her third child, she had noted an increase in the amount, duration, and frequency of menstrual flow. A dilatation and curettage (D & C) had been followed by a return to a normal cycle of twenty-seven days but with a heavy flow lasting four days. After this operation, she had received three transfusions of whole blood. Over the next several years, she had received eight additional blood transfusions. With the last two, she had developed hives, chills, fever, and symptoms of asthma. She had also taken vitamins and iron orally and had been given several injections of liver extract.

Gynecologists who examined her at the clinic found her to be obese, slow, somewhat dull, and apparently chronically ill. She was 66 inches in height and weighed 186 pounds. Her voice was husky and her skin was pale and dry. An electrocardiogram showed no abnormality of the heart. A test of thyroid function showed clear-cut hypothyroidism. Two months after she was placed on one and a half grains of thyroid daily, her menses returned to normal and all her other symptoms disappeared.

There isn't anything unique in the experience of this woman, not in the fact that low thyroid function was the cause of her menstrual disturbances as well as her other problems and not in the fact that her hypothyroidism went unrecognized for several years.

There are many possible causes for menstrual difficulties. Among them are ovarian cysts, fibroids, and cervical polyps. Endometriosis, a condition in which tissue like that found in the uterus occurs aberrantly in various locations in the pelvic cavity, can cause menstrual problems. But in the vast majority of women, there is no evidence of any organic problem. What is evident commonly if it is sought is low thyroid function.

That many menstrual irregularities are hypothyroid in origin was firmly established in the last century when thyroid deficiencies were first recognized. Forty years ago, after many years of successful use of thyroid therapy, leading gynecologists in this country and elsewhere were reporting that thyroid had cured more menstrual disorders than all other medications combined.

Unfortunately, that lesson seems to have been largely lost. Unless the commonly used but unreliable thyroid function tests point to thyroid deficiency, patients are either denied thyroid therapy or have the medication discontinued if some other doctor previously prescribed it. Symptoms may have been relieved by thyroid and may recur if the medication is stopped and disappear again if the therapy is resumed, yet some physicians are adamant unless the laboratory test is positive.

Not infrequently, there may be no suspicion of the possibility of thyroid involvement and no check at all for it. Recently, within a period of a few months, I saw three women who had undergone hysterectomies before the age of twenty-five for excessive bleeding. None had been suspected of having low thyroid function yet each had numerous other symptoms of the disorder—easy fatigability, dry skin, circulatory disturbances—which promptly disappeared with adequate thyroid therapy. The odds are high that needless surgery might have been avoided and these women could have raised families if hypothyroidism had been considered earlier.

Even from the Start

The normal woman begins her periods at about the age of twelve or thirteen, flows for four or five days, suffers no cramps, and repeats the cycle every twenty-six to thirty days. She should be able to become pregnant when she wishes to, go through nine months of gestation with little more than occasional discomfort, and should be able to deliver a healthy baby after a labor of several hours during which, in my opinion, she is entitled to some sedation. (Anyone can be trained to withstand pain and not complain about it, but the physician who teaches his patients that the pain of childbirth is all mental should, at least, so I believe, listen to himself say that and then have an eight-pound watermelon shoved through his anus; I wonder if he could then convince himself that pain is all mental.)

Low thyroid function is capable of disordering menses in many ways, begining even with affecting its onset. Paradoxical as it may seem, it is a fact that hypothyroidism may either hasten the onset or delay it. It may bring on menstruation several years before the usual time. In one case reported in the medical literature, the girl was only five years and two months old when flow started and by age nine had fully developed breasts and pubic hair. At that point, a disturbance of thyroid function was suspected and thyroid therapy not only stopped the precocious menstruation but also led to regression of breast size and loss of pubic hair. Later, menstruation and development followed at the normal time.

Among patients known to me personally, the youngest at onset of menses was eight. Her thyroid deficiency was not recognized until the age of twenty-two when I saw her for problems other than menstrual difficulties alone.

Her history revealed that after her first period occurred at the age of eight, she skipped three months but then continued to have periods at irregular intervals thereafter. All through her childhood and adolescence, she displayed other indications of thyroid deficiency: repeated respiratory infections, fatigue, frequent headaches. These symptoms responded to thyroid therapy, her menstrual cycles became smoother and subsequently she had two healthy babies.

In preparation for writing this book, I reviewed the records of 301 current hypothyroid women patients who had had some type of menstrual difficulty. In not all, by any means, had low thyroid function affected onset of menses. For eight, however, menstruation had begun at the age of nine, and for nineteen at the age of ten. On the other hand, for forty-three, menstruation had not begun until the age of fifteen or later.

The Build-Up of Evidence

Thyroid deficiency was associated with menstrual disturbances even before thyroid therapy became available.

About one hundred years ago, when thyroidectomy —removal of the thyroid gland—came into use to help patients threatened with strangulation by huge goiters, menstrual irregularities developed in many women after the operation. When the British Commission investigated 100 patients with myxedema in 1888, 37 women among them had menstrual irregulartites. Fifteen of the 69 married women among the patients reported miscarriages and only six children had been born after onset of myxedema.

As soon as thyroid became available in 1891 for therapy, there were reports of successful use of it in menstrual problems. Some patients who had ceased menstruation prematurely resumed it; some who had suffered from excessive flow benefited; many who had experienced painful cramps were relieved. It seemed that a new era of reproductive physiology was at hand. When, later, the basal metabolism test became available for checking on thyroid function, many women not previously suspected of being hypothyroid were treated successfully with thyroid for their menstrual problems.

Among the many reports of the effectiveness of thyroid therapy was one in 1939. It covered fifty women, aged sixteen to thirty-four, with menstrual irregularities, in all of whom there was evidence of reduced thyroid function. On thyroid therapy, more than 90 percent of those with painful menstruation were relieved, most of them completely. The results were fully as good in converting irregular periods to normal, regular ones. And in six of seven women with excessive menstrual flow, normal flow was established.

In 1949, I published a report on 143 women with menstrual disorders whom I had seen in my practice and for whom, after taking a thorough history and carrying out a complete physical examination including examination of the pelvis, I had prescribed thyroid therapy. These were women without evidence of fibroids, ovarian cysts, or any other organic disease. In some, a basal metabolism test indicated thyroid deficiency; in others, the basal temperature test was used.

Forty-eight of the women suffered from menstrual cramps. Only five failed to get some relief from thyroid therapy; thirty-five experienced complete relief.

Forty-five of the women had irregular cycles. Forty-three benefited, with the cycles becoming completely regular in forty-one.

Fifty women suffered from excessive bleeding. Two

failed to benefit; two improved somewhat; forty-six resumed periods with normal flow.

Many of the women who benefited from thyroid therapy provided added evidence that it was the thyroid which was responsible. These were the women who, upon being relieved of their problem, stopped taking medication only to return in a few months with their original complaints. Thyroid therapy again overcame their difficulties.

As I indicated in the 1949 report, thyroid therapy in these patients not only helped with their menstrual problems but also brought improvement in general health. Many of the women had complained of undue fatigue, of requiring more than the usual amount of sleep and yet of awakening tired, of being nervous, irritable, easily upset by insignificant incidents. These symptoms were relieved.

In the many years since that report, I have seen many hundreds of women with menstrual problems and with low thyroid function indicated by below-normal-range basal temperatures respond to thyroid therapy.

In that time, there have been reports from other physicians underscoring the association between menstrual disturbances and hypothyroidism. In one study of ten unselected myxedematous women, only two had normal menses. In another with patients with severe menorrhagia, or excessive flow, thyroid therapy corrected the menorrhagia.

In a study at the Mayo Clinic covering fifty consecutive young women with hypothyroidism, twenty-eight had menstrual disturbances. Abnormally profuse menses was a common disturbance; frequent bleeding between periods was another; in some cases, both problems were present. Thyroid therapy relieved the disturbances.

But the twofold problem remains: the need for recognition that low thyroid function very often can provoke menstrual problems, and the need for recognition, too, that hypothyroidism may be present despite laboratory tests suggesting it is not.

In their report on the study at the Mayo Clinic, Drs. Joseph C. Scott, Jr., and Elizabeth Mussey observed that a patient may be considered to be mildly hypothyroid by one physician and euthyroid (with normal thyroid function) by another on the basis of a single interview or test. "No single test or procedure," they emphasized, "will define the status of the thyroid gland. Furthermore, any combination of methods may lead to erroneous interpretation or to inconsistent results. The clinician must have the faculty of correlating the clinical appearance of the patient with the laboratory findings."

Certainly, this is true, and I would add only that, for reasons already noted in this book, the basal temperature test can be a guide, often more valuable than any laboratory test, to recognition of a hypothyroid state.

Miscarriages

One of the most tragic experiences for a woman is to lose her baby through miscarriage. For some women, the tragedy is repeated many times.

Among the 301 women in my current practice with a history of some type of menstrual difficulty, 164 had miscarriages. Some had only one but the "champion"—if that is a suitable term to use in such a connection—is a woman who was pregnant sixteen times and had only five live births. I first saw her when she was sixty-three, much too late to do anything about her reproductive physiology. But her whole history—not only of menstrual difficulties and miscarriages but of many other symptoms often associated with low thyroid function—suggests that she was an unrecognized hypothyroid who might have been spared her childbearing tragedies and much other trouble in her life if she had been treated as a hypothyroid.

Certainly, miscarriage is not invariably related to low thyroid function. There are many other possible causes. Yet soon after thyroid therapy first became available, it was found that patients with a history of miscarriages often had a history compatible with thyroid deficiency and that full-term pregnancies might follow treatment with thyroid.

I remember one of my earliest miscarriage patients. She was the wife of a psychiatrist and had been able to carry through to term three babies in the course of seven pregnancies. When I suggested that she might have a thyroid deficiency that could account for her miscarriages, she told me that she had actually been on thyroid several times in the past and when she got to feeling well would stop taking the thyroid. When, together, we went back over her childbearing history, we found that she had had her live babies during the times she was on thyroid and her miscarriages during the times she had chosen to stop taking thyroid.

Another patient I saw many years ago was a twenty-four-year-old woman who had miscarried once and was then well along in her second pregnancy. She had a history of irregular menstruation with severe cramps, along with other symptoms compatible with low thyroid function. Her basal temperature was low. I placed her on thyroid but it was too late for this pregnancy and shortly afterward she miscarried again. Thereafter, however, continuing on thyroid therapy regularly, she had four successful pregnancies.

Infertility

Millions of married couples—an estimated 10 percent of the total—are unwillingly childless, longing for but unable, seemingly, to raise a family.

Infertility has many possible causes—and, certainly, among them is thyroid deficiency. Animals thyroidectomized at an early age lack reproductive power. Baby rabbits whose thyroids are removed at the age of three weeks never mate. Cretinized female swine, in experiments I have carried out, have never come into detectable estrus.

The thyroid gland is intimately linked with reproduction although all the details of how are still not completely understood. It is known that the gland becomes enlarged in women at puberty and with pregnancy. Sexual depression was noted long ago in both men and women with myxedema.

Thyroid secretions in adequate amounts appear to be essential for the development of the egg and for proper ovarian secretions. If thyroid function is low, an egg may be discharged from an ovary but it may not be fertilizable or, if fertilized, may not be capable of nesting so that pregnancy is quickly aborted.

The medical literature is full of reports going back many years that provide evidence that thyroid medication, used when indicated, is one of the most helpful measures in the treatment of infertility in both men and women. And not infrequently it may be needed by both partners in an infertile marriage.

One case I remember very well involved, at first, a woman who for seventeen years had tried in vain to become pregnant. There had been many efforts by many physicians to help her. Among the many tests which had been performed, were the standard tests for thyroid function which indicated that hers was a normal thyroid. It was not normal, however, by the basal temperature test. I placed her on thyroid and that did much for her general health but it did not overcome the infertility problem.

Fortunately, I finally saw her husband. He came in because of dysentery. Even as he walked through the door, it was obvious that he was markedly hypothyroid. He had the myxedema look, his face swollen and mask-like. He moved slowly, seemed clumsy, spoke with a slow drawl. He suffered from headaches, needed ten hours of sleep a night, had always been susceptible to respiratory infections, and had had five serious attacks of pneumonia in a twelve-year period.

His basal temperature was 95.2 degrees. When he, too, was placed on the thyroid therapy he needed, his health and his whole appearance improved and several months later his wife conceived and in due course, at age thirty-nine, delivered a healthy first baby. She had another boy two years later.

Toxemia of Pregnancy

Toxemia, one of the potentially serious complications of pregnancy, fortunately does not occur often. It produces excessive fluid retention, high blood pressure, albumin in the urine and, in severe cases, convulsions and coma. As a rule, it occurs during the last three months of pregnancy and is more common in women who are pregnant for the first time.

Although little is known about the cause of toxemia, thyroid deficiency may well be a factor. For it is well established that pregnancy entails an increase in the need for thyroid hormone since new growth is taking place and the load on circulation is about 50 percent higher.

It seems likely that the extra stress of pregnancy may aggravate a previously mild hypothyroidism and at least in some cases could precipitate toxemia. Some evidence for this was presented years ago by investigators who found that administration of thyroid to women threatened with toxemia often prevented development of the condition.

It seems to me more than coincidence that in the many years when I was functioning as a general practitioner and it was necessary for me to engage in obstetrics, I encountered only a single case of toxemia. During this time, I was checking for thyroid function both before and during pregnancy and using thyroid therapy when the function was low.

The single case of toxemia occurred in a woman who first sought help for her pregnancy toward the end, coming in then because of headaches and excessive weight gain resulting from fluid retention. Her blood pressure was high and she was excreting large quantities of albumin. Her basal temperature was low and she was promptly started on thyroid but it was too late; only a few days later, she had to be admitted to hospital in convulsions. A Caesarean section was performed and both mother and baby survived. I have a strong suspicion that the toxemia could have been avoided if she had come in as soon as she became pregnant, allowing her thyroid deficiency to be detected and treated then.

D & C's and Hysterectomies

I want to emphasize, at the risk of seeming to be repetitious, that undetected and untreated thyroid deficiency can lead to needless surgery on the reproductive organs.

The most frequent operation is dilatation and curettage (D & C). With hormone imbalance, the lining of the uterus may thicken and there may be profuse and prolonged bleeding during menstruation. As a result of the blood loss, the patient is weakened, becomes anemic, and is much more susceptible to infections. Brief hospitalization and scraping away of the uterine lining relieves the condition but does nothing to correct the cause and often the original condition reappears and the procedure must be repeated. Finally, the need for repeated dilatations and curettages may make hysterectomy seem to be the answer.

Yet the odds are good that in many such cases hypothyroidism is present and its correction will return menstruation to normal. That surgery is unnecessary in many cases was pointed out a quarter of a century ago by Dr. J.H. Means, a Harvard authority on the thyroid. Excessive menstruation, he wrote, "may be sufficiently impressive in ordinary myxedema so that in several cases that have come to our attention, patients have actually had a dilatation and curettage for it when all they needed was desiccated thyroid for treatment."

Excessive menstruation can occur at any age, as demonstrated by two cases reported from the Mayo Clinic by Dr. Griff T. Ross and his associates. Both had been referred for surgery because of the profuse menstrual flow.

The first was a fifty-five-year-old woman who had received five blood transfusions the week before. She had been experiencing excessive flow for six months. Her history revealed that for more than three years she had suffered from increasing fatigue, dryness of the skin, puffiness of the face, and hoarseness, all suggesting hypothyroidism. Her basal metabolic rate, when it was finally taken, proved to be −22 percent. She was given three grains of thyroid daily. After five days, her bleeding stopped. She was discharged on two grains of thyroid daily. When she returned five months later for a checkup her fatigue, skin dryness, and other symptoms had disappeared, her menstrual periods were regular, and her basal metabolism was normal.

The second woman was thirty-five years old and had required transfusion after losing more than one-third of her blood from profuse menstrual flow over a seven-week period. Between her third and fourth child she had had three D & C's for pathological bleeding. Her facial edema, dry skin, sparse body hair, and a basal metabolism of -29 percent left no doubt of the diagnosis. On three grains of thyroid daily, her menstrual bleeding stopped on the seventh day. When she returned to the Mayo Clinic for a checkup four months later, all of the symptoms of thyroid deficiency were gone, her menstrual periods were regular and the flow normal, and her metabolism was normal.

In my own experience, no patient has required a hysterectomy for pathological bleeding unless uterine fibroids were present. If organic problems could be ruled out, as they could be in the great majority of cases, thyroid deficiency usually could be detected and treatment with thyroid solved the problem.

The need for other surgery may be minimized by adequate thyroid therapy in women with low thyroid function. Cysts on the ovary are common in such women and correction of the thyroid deficiency often eliminates the cysts.

Fibroid tumors have been rare in hypothyroid women who have been maintained on adequate thyroid therapy. It is possible to produce fibroids in experimental animals by injection of estrogens, and there is evidence of excess of estrogens in hypothyroid women. In hypothyroidism, there is increased activity of the pituitary gland aimed at trying to stimulate the thyroid to produce more hormone secretions, and the increased pituitary activity may spill over to affect the ovaries and increase their estrogen output.

"The Pill" and Thyroid Function

Birth control pills have been and remain generally satisfactory. Adverse reactions, however, have been noted in some women. The most serious is thrombophlebitis, the development of blood clot in the presence of inflammatory changes, usually in a leg vein.

Low thyroid function, as we have noted before, tends to make for sluggish blood circulation which may then result in a tendency for the blood to coagulate.

The only women whom I have seen with blood clots associated with use of oral contraceptives have been a few who were put on them without any thought being given to thyroid function and whose histories left little doubt that they needed thyroid therapy before the contraceptives were started.

A safe rule to follow is to check basal temperature before beginning use of oral contraceptives and if the basal temperature is low, thyroid therapy should be employed along with contraceptives.

The Heart of the Problem

From what has been said, it would appear that the possibility of thyroid deficiency should be considered, and if found, should be treated in any woman with a menstrual abnormality or a reproductive problem.

It was generally agreed that correction of thyroid deficiency solved many such abnormalities and problems —until about 1940. Some forty years ago, in an address before the Section of Obstetrics and Gynecology at the annual meeting of the American Medical Association, Dr. Jennings C. Litzenberg, a Minneapolis gynecologist, summarized the experience of many physicians. He noted that 30 percent of previously sterile women with low basal metabolisms conceived on thyroid therapy. He pointed to reports from the Mayo Clinic that about 70 percent of women with menstrual abnormalities improved on thyroid therapy and he quoted Dr. Robert Frank, a prominent New York gynecologist's emphatic declaration, that "The sole endocrine preparation that has proved itself of real value has been thyroid extract, which is of use in patients with lowered metabolism." About that time, too, Dr. Emil Novak of Johns Hopkins University, author of a textbook on gynecology, was noting that thyroid medication for sterility and miscarriage is often more efficacious than any other form of treatment.

Up to 1940, the only test for thyroid function was the basal metabolism. Some physicians used it when they suspected thyroid deficiency and many of those who did use it recognized its limitations and placed only a limited amount of faith in it. Other physicians did not use it at all because of its limitations. There was far greater reliance then than ever since on physical examination of the patient, on a careful check of history to pick up any clues to thyroid deficiency in the patient's symptoms and problems, and on the physician's clinical impression.

There was reliance, then, too, whenever there was a possibility that the patient could have low thyroid function, when the symptoms fit, regardless of what the not-too-reliable laboratory testing might indicate, on "try and see," on starting with a small dose of thyroid and watching for improvement or lack of it.

The results were admirable. There were mistakes, of course, but not many—and the moderate doses of thyroid used did no harm even when thyroid function was normal. But many hypothyroid patients received treatment they needed. If not all benefited with relief of menstrual or reproductive problems, a great many did and even among those who did not, few failed to improve in general health and have relief from other hypothyroid symptoms.

About 1940, the Protein Bound Iodine test for thyroid function came into use. It was to be followed by other laboratory tests to measure thyroid function. For thyroid conditions, the era of the laboratory had appeared.

The result was a pendulumlike swing to an extreme. Many physicians came to look upon the results of laboratory tests as absolutes. If a patient was hypothyroid, the laboratory was the place to determine so. If laboratory tests failed to indicate hypothyroidism, it could not be present—no matter the patient's symptoms or even if a patient was already on thyroid therapy and benefiting from it. Willy-nilly, if the lab report came back negative for low thyroid function, the patient got no thyroid therapy and if the patient was already on it he or she was taken off it.

It was to be years before there began to be recognition that the laboratory couldn't be the final arbiter. There began to be doubts about the value of the PBI test and, in 1967, Dr. Herbert Selenkow, Harvard thyroid specialist, crystallized them, pointing to PBI's many pitfalls and unreliability. Since then, other authorities have been pointing out that all commonly used lab tests for thyroid function leave much to be desired, that they are useful in some but not all cases, and that they are no substitute for a good physician's knowledge of what thyroid deficiency can bring about and his expert clinical impression of what it may be doing in the case of an individual patient.

I certainly hold no brief for the basal temperature as the ultimate test. But until something better comes along, it can, I know, help many physicians to help patients.

10

The Hypertension
Association

HYPERTENSION—high blood pressure—is a strange disease. It is potentially disabling, often fatal, exceedingly common, and long silent. It can be present for years without alerting its victims, giving them no clue to its presence, producing no identifying symptom.

Twenty-three million Americans, according to the National Heart and Lung Institute, have the disease. Yet half of those who have it don't know they have it, and half of those who know they have it are not being treated for it.

From scores of recent studies has come documentation of how much risk hypertension carries. Heart attacks are three to five times commoner in hypertensives than in others; stroke, four times commoner; congestive heart failure, five times commoner. The risk of potentially fatal kidney failure—and also of blindness—is increased. The higher the blood pressure, the greater the risk. But even mild elevation of pressure, left untreated, can shorten life, cutting seventeen years from the life expectancy of a thirty-five-year-old man, for example.

Hypertension is not reserved only for certain age groups or for certain types of people. It affects men and women of every national origin and at every age level. It affects young adults in their twenties as well as older people in their seventies and eighties. It affects teenagers and many children and has been found in four-year olds.

Currently, efforts are being made to mount an all-out campaign against hypertension. The U. S. Department of Health, Education and Welfare has launched a National Hypertension Information Program—an unprecedented cooperative effort involving all the health forces of the government, including the National Institutes of Health, the Food and Drug Administration, and the Health Services and Mental Health Administration, combined with the American Medical Association and organized medicine, and with industry and insurance and pharmaceutical companies—to fight the disease.

There are many possible causes of hypertension. Some are known; some are not. Is there ever an association between low thyroid function and hypertension? Can the correction of low thyroid function help to prevent hypertension? Can correction of hypothyroidism—mild, moderate, or severe—contribute to reducing already-present high blood pressure and possibly in some cases be enough in itself to restore the blood pressure to normal levels?

If correction of thyroid deficiency can help in the battle against hypertension, it would be an important dividend. And I believe it can help.

The System

Although blood pressure may seem mysterious, it isn't. It is simply the force, the push, against the walls of arteries as blood flows through them.

Each time the heart beats, pumping out blood, the pressure in the arteries of course increases; each time the heart relaxes between beats, the pressure goes down.

When a physician measures blood pressure, he makes two readings and writes them in the form of a fraction, for example, 130/80. The first and larger figure is the systolic pressure (when the heart beats) and the second is the diastolic pressure (when the heart rests).

It is entirely normal—and desirable—for pressure to fluctuate, to decrease during sleep, to increase during physical exertion or emotional excitement. The body's system for regulating blood pressure is a remarkable one, a finely tuned mechanism which, under normal circumstances, can adapt instantly to the shifting needs for blood of all organs and tissues.

During sleep, with the body in a horizontal position, there is less effect of gravity and less pressure is needed to get blood to the brain and so the pressure goes down. The pressure automatically goes up when the upright position is assumed in order to counter the gravity effect. And the pressure control system ordinarily works just as automatically and well to meet varying demands during work, play, eating, and under circumstances of fear, anger, and other emotions. But the control system can become impaired, resulting in chronic high blood pressure.

There is a wide range of normal blood pressure. At rest, a systolic pressure in the 100 to 140 range and a diastolic in the 60 to 90 range are considered normal. Nor does any single isolated reading above 140/90 indicate abnormal pressure. But when the elevation is continuous, hypertension has to be diagnosed.

The Stealth and the Damage

Hypertension is easy enough for a physician to discover through a simple test that takes only a minute or so and requires only wrapping a blood pressure cuff around one arm, applying a stethoscope, and taking a reading on a gauge. And rarely will anyone with hypertension be aware of its presence unless informed so by a physician. Hypertension can be present for years without producing any symptoms at all. Even when it does produce some symptoms—such as headache, dizziness, weakness, or fatigue—they may not be recognized for what they are since they are common to many other disorders.

But hypertension can be doing its potentially deadly work whether or not symptoms are present. When the heart must pump against excessive pressure, it must pump harder; there is a strain on it. To accommodate to the extra burden, the heart may enlarge and carry on well for years, but eventually the enlarged, overstretched heart muscle may weaken and heartbeat abnormalities may follow. Each year, about 50,000 Americans have been dying of such *hypertensive heart disease.*

Although it is serious enough, hypertensive heart disease is overshadowed by *coronary heart disease* with its heart attacks that strike 7,000 Americans a day and kill more than 600,000 a year.

If you put a garden hose under excessive pressure and keep it under such pressure for a long period of time, the hose becomes damaged. Similarly, excessive pressure in the coronary arteries that feed the heart muscle may damage the artery walls and provide sites at damaged points where materials carried in the blood may settle out and form deposits. Some investigators believe that excess pressure may even help to pound the deposits in and start the build-up which eventually narrows the bore of an artery, the channel through which blood can flow, thus reducing the flow to the heart muscle and paving the way for heart attack.

Since 1949, the community of Framingham, Massachusetts, has served as a vital experimental community. Investigators there have been following closely more than 5,000 men and women to determine which of them, healthy at the start, would develop heart disease and other problems, and why. And one result of that study has been the finding that heart attacks have been three to five times more common in Framingham residents with hypertension than in those without.

Not only does hypertension make a heart attack more likely but it also increases the deadliness when an attack occurs. The Health Insurance Plan of Greater New York has shown that among men with hypertension before a first heart attack, the number dead within thirty days after the attack is twice the number among men with normal pressure before the attack. Moreover, compared with men with normal pressure who survive a first attack, hypertensive men who survive have twice the risk of a second attack and more than five times the risk of death from heart attack during the next four and a half years.

The likelihood of stroke, too, is vastly increased by hypertension. That terrible disease—it was given its name centuries ago because of a belief that a victim was struck down by God—most commonly is caused by clogging deposits in brain arteries. Two million Americans today are living with stroke-caused disabilities: paralysis, loss of sensation, loss of balance, loss of vision, or loss of speech. And yearly, strokes kill at least 200,000 Americans.

The role of hypertension in strokes has been shown by many studies, including the Framingham study. The risk of strokes is five times higher among people with even moderately elevated (160/95) levels of blood pressure than among those with normal pressures.

Hypertension, too, has been found to be the principal reason for congestive heart failure. The failure develops when the heart's pumping power becomes so impaired that not enough blood is circulated to provide sustenance for all body tissues. The kidneys, suffering from lack of adequate circulation, no longer remove enough water from the blood, and urine output drops while the retained water accumulates in the lungs and other tissues. In the Framingham study, congestive heart failure proved to be five times as frequent among hypertensives as among people with normal blood pressure.

The Causes

Hypertension can occur at any age. In a survey in New Orleans, for example, the incidence of elevated pressure was 54 percent among people over the age of fifty, but even at ages twenty to twenty-nine 6 percent were affected; at ages thirty to thirty-nine, 16 percent, and at ages forty to forty-nine, 35 percent. In a Georgia study, 11 percent of teen-agers had high blood pressure. At Washington University School of Medicine, hypertension has been found in four-year-old children.

What causes hypertension?

In only 10 to 15 percent of all cases can some definite physical cause be found. It may be a narrowing (coarctation) of the aorta, the great artery that emerges from the heart and from which other arteries of the body branch off. This type of hypertension can be cured by surgery to eliminate the narrowed portion of the aorta.

In some cases, a tumor of the adrenal gland, called a pheochromocytoma, may be responsible. The tumor is usually benign but it produces excess quantities of materials that elevate blood pressure. Such hypertension, too, is curable by surgery to remove the tumor.

In some cases, obstruction to normal blood flow in a kidney artery produces high blood pressure. Many years ago, at Western Reserve University, experiments in which a clamp was applied to restrict flow through the kidney arteries of animals showed that if the flow was reduced moderately, mild high blood pressure developed and with a greater flow reduction severe hypertension developed.

This work paved the way for the discovery that a protein material called renin, which is liberated by a blood-starved kidney, acts chemically in the blood to trigger pressure elevation. Such work helped to explain the influence of the artery disease, atherosclerosis, with its clogging deposits, on blood pressure in some cases. If atherosclerosis affects a kidney artery, the reduction of blood flow can cause release of renin by the kidney as effectively as a clamp.

But the vast majority of hypertensive cases—85 to 90 percent of the total—have been considered to be essential or idiopathic, meaning that no definite physical cause for them could be found. They can be treated effectively in most instances with any one or several of a wide variety of drugs now available to lower blood pressure even though these drugs do not get at whatever may be causing the elevation.

Meanwhile, however, evidence has been accumulating for many years that the thyroid gland may play a role in hypertension. Unfortunately, the evidence has been neglected by most students of hypertension and even by investigators in the field of thyroid physiology. Dr. Sidney C. Werner, a senior author of a recent medical book, *The Thyroid* (Harper & Row, 1971), dismisses the hypothyroid-hypertension connection in a single sentence: "In hypothyroidism, blood pressure is often elevated to hypertensive levels of systolic and diastolic pressures, returning to normal after treatment." Such successful reduction of elevated pressure certainly warrants further consideration.

The Link

In retrospect, it is probably highly significant that the first case of thyroid deficiency autopsied by Dr. W.M. Ord in England about a century ago showed kidney damage and marked kidney artery atherosclerosis.

Half a century ago, Dr. A.M. Fishberg, a New York City clinician, pointed to the role of hypothyroidism in artery disease. He cited in *The Journal of the American Medical Association* the case of a twenty-one-year-old man who had died of pneumonia. He had been free of any seemingly serious illness prior to the pneumonia but his blood pressure had been high: 175/135. On autopsy, his thyroid gland was found to be almost completely nonfunctioning; it had been largely replaced by fatty tissue. He had generalized atherosclerosis which had affected the kidney arteries as well as other arteries of the body. There was reason to believe that the impairment of circulation to the kidneys had led to the hypertension and Dr. Fishberg suggested that the hypothyroidism and atherosclerosis in this man were closely related.

I became interested in the possible association between hypothyroidism and hypertension in 1958 when I spent some time studying goiter patients at the Kaiserin Elizabeth Hospital in Vienna. These patients had much higher blood pressures than did my patients back in the United States. They displayed a gradual rise in pressure with age. What was striking, too, was that some of these goiter patients who had needed several operations —partial thyroid removals—to prevent the choking threatened by their greatly enlarged glands experienced an increase in blood pressure with each successive operation. Apparently, the more thyroid gland removed, the higher the pressure went.

When I returned home, I checked the case records of all patients who had been placed on thyroid therapy during the previous ten years.

The Record and an Instructive Case

Among the patients placed on thyroid during the ten-year period, ninety-five had been hypertensive in varying degrees. Of the ninety-five, only five had failed to show satisfactory declines in pressure after being placed on thyroid therapy.

Only a few months later, a myxedematous patient walked into the office and provided a demonstration of the role of neglected thyroid deficiency in hypertension.

She was then thirty-eight years old and the past seven years had been turbulent ones for her. Her early history had been uneventful. She had been married at age nineteen and had had two successful pregnancies, the first of which yielded twin boys and the second a girl. Her troubles began in August 1951 when she was hospitalized because of inflammation of leg veins. Her blood pressure at that time was 140/90. She recovered from the inflammation.

Her next hospitalization was in April 1952 for hysterectomy because of a fibroid tumor. Her blood pressure then was 128/90. Four months later, she was readmitted to the hospital, this time because of extreme nervousness and shakiness. Her blood pressure then was 130/99 and her basal metabolism rate was normal.

There was no medical consultation. The surgeon, evidently convinced that the basal metabolism test result was not valid and that her nervousness and shakiness were due to excessive thyroid activity (and evidently, too, overlooking the likelihood that her premature menopause might have had something to do with them), performed a thyroidectomy. The pathologist's report on the removed thyroid tissue indicated it was normal, not diseased, tissue.

Eleven months later she was hospitalized again for removal of her gall bladder. Now her blood pressure was 160/100. Over the next two and a half years, her hypertension became more severe and failed to respond to measures prescribed by several physicians. In March 1957 she was hospitalized for adrenal gland exploration. Her blood pressure was 190/130. A kidney cyst and half of the left adrenal gland were removed without effect on the blood pressure and she was readmitted six weeks later for partial removal of the right adrenal, again without improvement.

I saw her in December 1958—with a blood pressure of 200/130 and full-blown myxedema. She was started on one grain of thyroid daily and over the next several weeks, her blood pressure began to come down a little. Three months later, she was taking two grains of thyroid daily and her blood pressure was down to near-normal level. Her thyroid dosage was then raised to three grains.

Her blood pressure became normal and she went to work to help out with her family's strained finances.

She continued to work for the next six years. A move to another city occasioned a change in physicians and the new one stopped the thyroid medication and placed her on diuretics and tranquilizers.

When I saw her in my office again in December 1971, six years after her last visit, her blood pressure was again way up, 200/130. Her cholesterol level which had been 207 on thyroid therapy was up to 356. During the six years, she had developed arthritis which had become so severe that she had become addicted to pain pills.

The diuretics and tranquilizers were stopped and thyroid therapy reinstituted. Gradually the blood pressure came down to 150/100 but remained at this level. She was still taking pain pills. She was found dead eighteen months later and at first suicide was suspected. The autopsy revealed severe kidney artery atherosclerosis and it is probable that impaired kidney function allowed accumulation of the pain medication in her body and her death was accidental.

Her case resembles that of the young man described by Dr. Fishberg many years ago but in this case two courses of thyroid therapy brought the hypertension down to normal or near-normal levels. There seems little doubt that the thyroidectomy had much to do with her hypertension, triggering it or at the very least aggravating it.

More Experience

As I began to pay increasing attention to cases of hypertension, my notice was drawn to reports from

South Africa by Dr. Pericles Menof that thyroid therapy was efficacious. His practice was to begin treatment with five grains and then reduce the dosage as indicated.

It seemed to me that better results might be obtained by starting with small doses and increasing them gradually if necessary. Nevertheless, Menof reported that many of his hypertensive patients improved. Patients whose hypertension was due to kidney disease, however, did not benefit from thyroid therapy, Menof found, and this has been my experience as well. If the kidney artery becomes atheromatous and clogged, thyroid therapy could not be expected to improve the circulation to the kidney.

I have seen many patients with hypertension—mild, moderate and even severe—respond to thyroid therapy. One twenty-five-year-old man first seen in 1967 had been refused by the military at the age of twenty because of his elevated blood pressure. He had been hospitalized then while a careful search for kidney involvement was made. There was no such involvement and he was placed on antihypertensive medication.

Perhaps the medication was ineffective; perhaps he was not very conscientious about taking it, either out of forgetfulness or because of undesirable side effects. On his first visit to me, I found his blood pressure to be quite high, 200/100. I noted symptoms suggestive of hypothyroidism, including dry skin and tendency to undue fatigue. Previous testing of thyroid function, including a PBI test, had indicated normal thyroid function. But his basal temperature was low.

Because he was a big man weighing 219 pounds, he was started on two grains of thyroid daily. Later this was raised to four grains. It took several weeks before his pressure began to come down at all and many months before it came all the way down. But down it did come, without use of any other medication, to reach a highly desirable level of 130/80.

The incidence of hypertension may be as high as one in ten and of hypothyroidism, four in ten. Both conditions tend to be familial. Unless the hypothyroidism protected against hypertension, one would expect some overlapping, with both conditions occurring together in the same individual in many cases. The evidence indicates that instead of protecting against it, low thyroid function may promote elevation of blood pressure.

Evidence of the value of correcting low thyroid function in combating hypertension also comes from a heart disease followup study I have had in progress since 1950. It has covered more than 1,500 patients placed on thyroid therapy for hypothyroidism and followed for many years. The aim of the study, to begin with, was to determine what influence the correction of low thyroid function might have on heart disease. (We shall be considering the findings in terms of heart disease in some detail in a later chapter.) The study has also provided opportunity to determine on a fairly substantial scale the influence of thyroid therapy on hypertension.

The incidence of hypertension among these patients when they entered the study was about 10 percent, about the same as generally accepted estimates of the incidence in the general population. Over the years, only twelve new cases of hypertension have appeared among the patients in the study. Yet many more were to be expected since the incidence of hypertension increases with age. In the general population, to age twenty-four, 10.9 percent of men and 1.4 percent of women have elevated blood pressure. By age fifty-four, 15.3 percent of women and 17.7 percent of men are hypertensive. By age sixty-four, the incidence is 24.3 percent for women and 27.5 percent for men.

Thus, patients on thyroid therapy had marked protection against the development of elevated blood pressure if they did not already have it when they entered the study, and in the vast majority of those who were hypertensive when they entered, thyroid therapy alone, without antihypertensive medication, was enough to bring down the blood pressure.

All told, only seven patients have required antihypertensive medication in addition to thyroid therapy. One of these is a woman first seen years ago when she was fifty-three. She had had hypertension for five years and had been treated for it with antihypertensive drugs. In spite of the medication, she had a blood pressure of 165/90 when first seen. She also had chest pain on walking, a high cholesterol level of 380, and was thyroid deficient.

She was placed on thyroid and the antihypertensive medication was stopped. Her cholesterol level came down to 250 and her blood pressure to 150/80 and for ten years she did fine except for a period of time when the thyroid therapy was interrupted. She lived at a distance, in another state. I did not see her between 1969 and 1972. During those years, her local doctor took her off thyroid therapy and put her on antihypertensive medication again. When she returned in 1972, her blood pressure was 170/100. Again she was placed on thyroid therapy and the antihypertensive medication was discontinued, and her blood pressure came down to 150/80.

Recently, however, thyroid therapy alone has not been enough to control her blood pressure. She is now on both thyroid and antihypertensive medication and the combination is maintaining the control. I suspect that her kindey arteries now have been affected by her atherosclerosis, which was advanced enough when she started thyroid therapy to be causing chest pain, and the hypertensive effects of the kidney artery disease can't be overcome by the thyroid therapy alone.

Another patient for whom thyroid therapy failed to control hypertension was fifty-eight when she was first seen. She had suffered from hypertension for many years and in spite of treatment for it her blood pressure was 160/90. She was hypothyroid and her history indicated that she had been for much of her life. Her menstrual periods had not begun until she was sixteen. She was never regular and after a miscarriage was sterile. She had frequent respiratory infections including a severe attack of bilateral pneumonia, suffered from severe migraine headaches, and had periods of depression. On thyroid therapy, the depressions cleared, the headaches seldom occurred, and she felt so much better that she refused to take antihypertensive medicine. For seven years her blood pressure stayed at about 150/90 on thyroid therapy alone, but then it began to rise.

She refused other medication and at times the pressure would reach 180/100, but she felt well. She finally died at age seventy-four and the autopsy revealed generalized atherosclerosis with obstruction in the coronary arteries. Thyroid therapy had not completely controlled her hypertension although for a time it did so as well as antihypertensive drugs, and she felt much better without the migraine and depression. The tragic thing was that she was denied relief from thyroid deficiency early in her life. I can't be certain but I feel reasonably sure that the hypertension might have been avoided if she had been started on thyroid at an early age.

Of course, not all cases of hypertension by any means are related to thyroid deficiency. There are other known causes of blood pressure elevation and, undoubtedly, others that will become known.

But it seems to me to be obviously desirable that whenever there is any evidence of low thyroid function, it should be tested for, particularly since the basal temperature test is so simple and without cost. And if hypothyroidism is found, it should be treated at once and the treatment should be continued for life unless there is good reason to stop. Certainly, other symptoms of hypothyroidism will disappear and there is a good chance that hypertension may be avoided if it is not already present and controlled if it is an existing problem.

II

The Thyroid and Heart Attacks

INVESTIGATIONS OF MEDICAL MYSTERIES can be very much like those in fictional murder mysteries. First, one character becomes suspect, then another, and another, and another. The web of circumstantial evidence may seem almost complete. The suspects may look very much like murderers. Yet, in the end, the real criminal turns out to be someone previously unsuspected.

Of suspected culprits behind heart attacks, seemingly likely causes of the coronary artery disease that leads to the attacks, there has certainly been no shortage. They have been highly publicized; you are undoubtedly aware of them and, quite likely, worried about them. But do they solve the mystery? Do they even begin to tell the whole story?

I think you will be able to see for yourself, clearly, why they do not, why there has been so much confusion, and what it is that has been missing and that can clear up the

155

confusion and open the way immediately for use of a simple, practical measure to help cut greatly into the toll of heart attacks.

A Radical Change

Within the memory of millions now living, heart attack has risen from obscurity to become our deadliest predator. It now kills more than 600,000 Americans each year and disables many more. But it was no such threat only a few generations ago. Just since the 1930s, the death rate from heart attack has quadrupled.

Heart attack strikes some young people—in their twenties and thirties. At age forty, the annual rate of new attacks is about 3 per 1,000 among American men. At age fifty, 1 of every 100 men will develop coronary heart disease in the course of a year. Before age sixty, 1 of every 5 men will have the disease—and in most cases a heart attack will be the first overt sign.

And although the magnitude of the problem for men has somewhat obscured its importance for women, in one recent year heart attacks accounted for 212,000 deaths among American women, a toll 60 percent greater than that from cancer.

What we have is an epidemic of a disease that was a relative rarity before this century. Something must have changed radically.

Saturated Fats and Cholesterol

As you well know, they have been blamed. But is the blame justified?

It's doubtful that saturated fats and cholesterol-rich foods make up any greater part of the diet of many people today than they did of the diet of our forefathers of one and two centuries ago.

Back then, much of the population lived on farms. Fresh dairy products and eggs were plentiful—and plentifully consumed. In winter, meat could be preserved and fat meat was far more palatable than tough, lean meat. In summer, cured bacon and hams were supplemented with pork sausage fried down in lard. Butter then was spread thickly on breakfast hot biscuits and on bread. From milk cooled in the old springhouse, thick cream was skimmed and used on fresh or canned fruit. I can remember well a saying of my grandfather: "Even shoe leather would taste good with cream and sugar on it."

If a high-fat, high-cholesterol diet were as dangerous as alleged, it would seem that just about every farmer in those days should have died of a heart attack, leaving the rest of the world to starve to death. But farmers were not dying of heart attacks a century or two ago.

Other Changes

Our sugar consumption is up and some scientists theorize that increased sugar intake may elevate certain blood fats, triglycerides, contributing to coronary artery disease. But convincing evidence of a link between sugar consumption and heart attacks is lacking.

Our coffee consumption is up and some studies have seemed to indicate that excess coffee drinking may be a bad influence on the heart, but other studies have failed to confirm such an influence. We may be drinking much more alcohol than our ancestors did, but the effect of alcohol on the heart is still not clearly established.

Our drinking water has come under suspicion—in particular, soft water, not in and of itself but because it may dissolve certain harmful minerals out of household plumbing.

The air we breathe has undergone vast changes in the last century and certainly air pollution from industry and from the automobile is not conducive to health. There is some evidence that carbon monoxide from automobile exhausts may contribute to heart problems. And cigarette smoke has been indicted as a possible factor in heart disease as well as in lung cancer.

Modern technology has reduced our physical labor at work and physical effort required getting to and from work. There are some who blame our sedentary way of life for the increase in heart attacks. The greatest enthusiast for vigorous exercise I have ever known was my college professor of physical education, a near-perfect model of a physical specimen, who had a heart attack before the age of fifty.

And there is, of course, stress, which is supposed to be much greater in modern society than ever before. And yet I wonder if it really is. Past generations had their stresses—their daily problems, often quite harsh, along with acute crises and disasters which were hardly any less frequent than today.

Of the many changes that have occurred, some may be contributing to the rise in mortality from heart attacks. But one change—a monumental one—has had little attention.

Clues in the Graz Autopsies

Death is a constant. If more people now are dying of heart attacks, of what did their counterparts die of before? There is something of great significance to be unearthed through a study of changing death patterns —and there is unique place for such a study.

Graz, Austria, is a unique location for the purpose for several reasons. First, only the Landeskrankenhaus is available for routine hospitalization, thus insuring that its patients are a cross-section of society in a city of 230,000 population, Austria's second largest. Second, a law passed by the renowned Empress Maria Theresa over two hundred years ago requires autopsy for all hospital deaths in the city. Third, the population is relatively stable, without major disruption in hundreds of years. Fourth, the diet and technologic development are comparable to those in the United States. The "iron age" was born near Graz over 2,000 years ago.

Each year, over 2,000 autopsies are performed in Graz, covering 75 percent of the total deaths in the city. The autopsy records show the cause of death in each case, and the records go back many years.

I have spent at least one month each summer for the past fifteen years reviewing autopsy records in Graz and in that time have examined more than 70,000!

One result is a medical report published in 1974 in *The Journal of the American Geriatrics Society* with the collaboration of Professor Max Ratzenhofer, head of the Pathological Institute of Graz, and Richard Gisi, a senior medical student who helped with the collection of critical data during the summer of 1973.

We made a comparison of the causes of death for two years—1930 and 1970. We chose those years because both were somewhat removed from wars which can materially affect death patterns.

Since, obviously, a rise in deaths from heart attacks could occur only if deaths from some other diseases declined, we divided all of the deaths for each year into four categories: those due to infections, those due to malignant diseases, those due to degenerative diseases, and those due to accidents and miscellaneous causes.

It became apparent that the most striking change during the forty-year interval was the reduction in deaths from infectious diseases. In 1930, almost half of all deaths were caused by infection. By 1970, there had been a 56 percent drop in such deaths. The decline began at the end of World War II when antibiotics became available.

Prior to the antibiotics, deaths from infection not only had been high but had occurred at early ages. In 1930, only 47 percent of the deaths were in people over age fifty. Fewer people lived to ages when they might be subject to diseases of later life. Heart attacks were rare; they accounted for 6.8 deaths per 1,000 autopsies in contrast to 426 deaths from infections per 1,000 autopsies.

By 1970, as a result of the drop in fatalities from infections, 67 percent of the total deaths were in patients over fifty years of age. This 20 percent rise in deaths at later years could be expected to increase the number of candidates eligible for heart attacks to some extent but it could *not* account for the huge jump in incidence. Between 1930 and 1970, deaths from heart attacks increased by a phenomenal 1,000 percent.

Either something new had entered the picture to cause

the increase *or those surviving premature deaths from infections were prone to develop heart disease*. Careful study of the autopsy protocols indicated that the latter was true.

In 1930, tuberculosis was, as it had been for a century, the leading cause of death. It continued to be until the coming of the antibiotics in 1945. Then, between 1945 and 1970, deaths from tuberculosis plummeted. The decline in tuberculosis deaths accounted for 63 percent of the total decline in deaths from infectious diseases.

That meant that the odds were almost two to one that individuals contributing to a rise in deaths from degenerative or malignant diseases in 1970 were those who had escaped death from tuberculosis. The rise in heart attacks had been 1,000 percent, much greater than the rise in malignancies. In only twenty-five years, deaths from tuberculosis had been traded for deaths from heart attack, which had become the new champion killer.

The Drop and the Rebound

During World War II, heart attacks dropped all over Europe. And in Graz, as well, although heart attacks were rare in 1939, the incidence fell an additional 75 percent by 1944.

The reduction in heart attacks during the war has been ascribed to a war-caused change in diet, notably a reduction in cholesterol—and saturated fat-rich foods. And there is no question that diet did change during the war.

The same change in diet took place in Graz as elsewhere. But a review of the autopsies carried out in Graz during World War II shows that although heart attacks dropped 75 percent during the war years, coronary atherosclerosis—the choking up of the coronary arteries that leads to heart attacks—was more severe than before.

The mystery was: What unknown factor had lowered the heart attack death rate in the face of a rising rate of severe coronary atherosclerosis? The answer was simple when the categories of death causes for the years 1939 and 1944 were compared in the autopsy records. The war had caused a great rise in deaths from tuberculosis and other infectious diseases—and these had removed persons afflicted with accelerating coronary atherosclerosis before heart attack could occur. The autopsy reports showed that the coronary arteries of patients dying of tuberculosis were so diseased that they would have had a heart attack if tuberculosis had not won the race.

Each country in Europe that showed a drop in heart attacks during the war showed a marked rise in infectious deaths, including those from tuberculosis. It would seem that death from tuberculosis or another infectious disease is a far more powerful deterrent to heart attack than the alleged influence of diet.

As soon as specific drugs for tuberculosis became available, deaths from this disease dropped sharply. The next year, heart attacks began to rise.

And autopsy studies of the coronary arteries in those dying of tuberculosis and of the lungs of those dying of heart attacks left no doubt about the close relationship of the two diseases. Patients over sixty years of age dying of tuberculosis had far-advanced coronary atherosclerosis, and heart attacks were imminent. When deaths from tuberculosis decreased, patients dying of heart attacks had tuberculosis in their lungs.

It was evident why heart attacks had replaced tuberculosis as the leading cause of death. The same patient was susceptible to both diseases—and as soon as he could escape death from tuberculosis and survive into the later years, heart attack took over as the new enemy.

An Answer to the Mystery

One of the great puzzles about heart attacks can be understood now on the basis of the relationship between tuberculosis and coronary disease and the insight that heart attacks are occurring in a "new population" made up of those who have escaped earlier death from tuberculosis.

Throughout the world, there have been more deaths from heart attacks among men than among women. Vast sums and much research effort have gone into trying to find the reason why. For a time some investigators felt that the female sex hormones were providing some protection for women. Attempts were made to administer female hormones to men who had survived a first heart attack in hope of preventing further damage. However, a need almost to wear brassieres and a loss of sexual drive did not seem worthwhile to most men. Moreover, when the Veterans Administration began to use female hormones to delay cancer of the prostate, it was found that atherosclerosis became a major problem. The female hormone offered no protection.

Now, in the light of the tuberculosis-heart attack relationship, consider that, for some unknown reason, the male has always been more susceptible to several infectious diseases, and this is particulary true of tuberculosis.

In all of the countries reporting to the World Health Organization, there is a preponderance of males afflicted with tuberculosis. WHO statistics show for the years 1947–1949, for example, the death rate from tuberculosis per 100,000 population for Japan was 169 for males and 129 for females; for Italy, 59 males and 38 females; for England, 53 males and 33 females; for Canada, 34 males and 28 females; and for the United States, 30 males and 14 females.

The preponderance of males in death from tuberculosis is similar to that in deaths from heart attacks. If the rise in heart attacks stems from elimination of premature deaths from tuberculosis, then there are more male candidates for heart attacks available. The reason for the increased susceptibility of the male to infectious diseases must be left for future study.

But Why the Young?

Although heart attacks are the leading cause of death at present, their rise has not signaled the fall of civilization. In reality, man is living longer than at any time in history and may be suffering less from pain and disability.

As long as tuberculosis ruled the roost, death usually came before age forty, and only after many months spent in bed with racking cough, weakness, and wasting. The average age of death from heart attack in Graz is sixty-six years and often there is no history of illness until the fatal attack.

Death from heart attack, when it comes suddenly at the end of a morbidity-free, productive, and happy normal life-span, is a humane type of death. But it does not, of course, always come suddenly. Heart attacks may strike repeatedly in the same individual before they finally kill, producing invalidism in the interim. And they too often strike the middle-aged and the young.

An attempt to study young patients with heart attacks was made in 1946 by the late famed cardiologist Dr. Paul Dudley White and a Harvard colleague, Dr. Jacob Lerman. Their interest was aroused by reports of heart attacks in young men during World War II. Among American military personnel, 866 men aged eighteen to thirty-nine had experienced heart attacks.

Drs. White and Lerman investigated twenty-eight men who had survived a heart attack before the age of forty. They found that two abnormalities stood out clearly: serum cholesterol was high and the basal metabolism rate was usually low.

Thyroid therapy was tried cautiously and some improvement was noticed. The cholesterol levels fell; the patients felt better; those with anginal pain, the chest pain associated with coronary artery disease, became pain-free with only two exceptions, and none of those without angina developed the pain during treatment.

These results were neglected for years. It was not until 1960 that I encountered the report and promptly wrote to Dr. White, asking him why he had never published further on this subject. He replied that after a time the cholesterol levels in the men had started to rise again, and he had decided that thyroid therapy might be a blind alley and had sought other answers. But the last sentence of Dr. White's letter indicated what the problem had been; in it, he noted that the dosages of thyroid used had been in the range of just one-tenth to one-quarter of a grain daily—very minute dosages, hardly likely to suffice.

Had Dr. White been as versed in thyroid physiology as he was in cardiology, we might long ago have had a broad medical profession and public awareness of the role of the thyroid in coronary artery disease and heart attacks.

Actually, twelve years before, Dr. L.M. Hurxthal at the Lahey Clinic in Boston had clearly shown that thyroid secretion controls the cholesterol level in most patients. In patients with hyperthyroidism, or excessive thyroid activity, he had found, the cholesterol level in the blood was below the average normal level. After surgery on the excessively active thyroid gland, the cholesterol level climbed above normal if too much thyroid tissue had been removed, making the patient hypothyroid. But then, if the hypothyroid patient were given the proper dosage of thyroid, the cholesterol level fell into the normal range and stayed there. If only Dr. White had adjusted his thyroid dosages to meet the needs of his patients! But Dr. White was caught up in the tide of epidemiological investigations of environmental factors that might be involved in heart attacks and spent much of the rest of his life, when he was not treating patients, in such investigations.

Before looking at the striking evidence that thyroid deficiency is the most potent factor in the development of atherosclerosis and heart attacks, it will be well to recount the evidence that misled Dr. White and many other scientists for many years into believing that nothing else will do except changing our mode of living to conquer heart disease.

Since cholesterol has been a core factor in that argument, we need to know some of the interesting facts about this most interesting compound in order to evaluate the evidence.

The Matter of "Solid Bile"

Cholesterol was discovered by a French chemist more than two hundred years ago in the course of a study of gallstones. The flaky, white crystalline material is insoluble in water but dissolves readily in chloroform, ether, and other fat solvents. Because of its origin, it was given the name "cholesterol"—from the Greek meaning "solid bile."

Over the years, it has been established that cholesterol is found only in animals, not plants. Along the borderline between animal and plant organisms, some forms of life contain the substance while others do not. Most bacteria, for example, do not contain cholesterol but the colon bacillus, a bacterium native to the intestinal tract, does contain small quantities.

In mammals, not only is cholesterol to be found in every cell but also present in each cell are enzymes for the local production of the compound when needed. Obviously, cholesterol must be a vital material or these enzymes would disappear.

In humans, at the time of birth, even the brain contains the enzymes for producing cholesterol and as a child develops much more cholesterol is added to the central

nervous system. However, in the adult, there is no replacement of cells in the brain and spinal cord, and the
enzymes disappear from these tissues. All other tissues in
the body replace worn or damaged cells, and the enzymes
necessary for production of cholesterol remain throughout life.

Like other herbivorous animals, the human who is a
strict vegetarian, gets no cholesterol in his diet yet his
tissues and blood contain the normal amount of cholesterol. Apparently, the production enzymes are capable of
forming all the cholesterol that is needed.

On the other hand, carnivorous animals and non-
vegetarian humans get large quantities of cholesterol in
their diets. If too much cholesterol accumulates in the
blood, the liver normally breaks down some of the excess
into bile salts which are excreted in the bile. Attempts to
lower levels of cholesterol in the blood through fat-free
diets or use of polyunsaturated fats may have only a
temporary effect since enzymes of the body will synthesize more cholesterol as need arises.

Cholesterol can be formed from the simplest foods,
whether they are carbohydrates, proteins, or fats. Only a
molecule containing two carbon atoms is necessary for
the start of the formation of the complex cholesterol
molecule that contains four benzene rings and a side
chain. The rapid synthesis of cholesterol is, in fact, one of
nature's wonders. It appears that by making it possible to
start synthesis with simple building blocks nature
guarantees that cholesterol will always be available when
needed, and a necessary material it is in many ways.

The hen's egg is rich in cholesterol because the material is required if a chick is to develop. In the human body,

the adrenal glands contain the highest concentration of cholesterol of any tissues in the body. Cholesterol is the starting material for the synthesis of adrenal hormones needed for the maintenance of mineral and glucose metabolism and to ready the body for quick action in emergency situations.

Although the brain and spinal cord account for only 2 percent of total body weight, they contain almost one-fourth of the total cholesterol in the body. Some of this is present in supportive connective tissue but some is believed to serve as insulation for nerve fibers. The skin is also rich in cholesterol, containing about 10 percent of total body stores. Sunlight converts this cholesterol to vitamin D, essential to bone metabolism and prevention of rickets.

Cholesterol is also to be found in the marrow within bones where blood cells are formed. As it is for the adrenal gland hormones, it is also the starting point for sex hormones.

It is hardly surprising that, since cholesterol is so essential in the body, an attempt a few years ago to lower cholesterol levels in the blood by interfering with synthesis of the compound in the body led to blindness and death.

A Whirl of Confusion

Since cholesterol is such an essential body material, how could it have become suspected as a culprit in causing premature disease of the arteries and heart attacks?

The story begins in 1858, long before heart attacks

were recognized. Rudolph Virchow, professor of pathology in Berlin and the father of the new science of pathology, demonstrated that when tissue degenerated, large amounts of cholesterol were liberated. This fact has been remembered but something even more important that Virchow demonstrated was forgotten. He clearly showed that cholesterol did not cause the damage to the tissue but rather was released as a result of the damage.

Repeatedly in the last one hundred years, other pathologists have confirmed the observations of Virchow: Cholesterol is not present in abnormal amounts at the beginning of degenerative processes, only after the processes are well along.

Nevertheless, attention began to be focussed on cholesterol as a culprit when, fifty-five years after Virchow's work, a Russian physiologist, N. Anitschkow, reported that when he stuffed rabbits with cholesterol, he got changes in their arteries somewhat similar to those appearing in the arteries of patients suffering from heart attacks. It seemed to Anitschkow that there was a cause and effect relationship.

There were to be objections to Anitschkow's conclusions on many grounds. Rabbits are vegetarians and never eat cholesterol-containing foods; as a result, they are not adapted to eliminating excess cholesterol and so their blood values of cholesterol when fed it in excess are high. No such elevations occur nor does damage to the arteries develop in other animals—rats and dogs, for example—on similar feedings.

As investigators followed in Anitschkow's footsteps, some were able to show that even these animals could be made to develop atherosclerosis if they were fed in the laboratory huge amounts of cholesterol, far greater than what the animals would consume normally outside the laboratory. Moreover, the levels to which cholesterol in the blood had to be raised were no less unrealistic.

For example, in cholesterol feeding experiments with dogs, the blood cholesterol level had to be raised to 4,000 and higher before atherosclerosis developed, but outside the laboratory a blood cholesterol level of 400 in man or dog is considered very high.

Even beyond this, some scientists recently have scrutinized the animal feeding experiments done in the past in the light of important new knowledge. They have found that in none of the experiments were the animals fed the large amounts of cholesterol in the form in which it occurs naturally in food but instead in the form of crystalline cholesterol or heat-dried egg yolk powder. And the chow was made up in large batches to last many days or weeks.

And that makes a vital difference. Once such crystalline or powdered cholesterol is exposed to air, it is changed chemically to form other compounds, some of which are injurious to the linings of arteries.

A significant discovery of modern research is that when an artery lining is normally healthy, cholesterol in the blood moves in and out of the lining, but when the lining is damaged, cholesterol can move in more readily than it can move out, and this happens even when blood cholesterol levels are entirely normal.

And in very recent animal experiments in which crystalline cholesterol or heat-dried egg yolk powder has been used, investigators have detected signs of artery damage within just a few days, well before cholesterol levels in the blood even had a chance to rise above normal.

It thus appears that not cholesterol feeding but rather feeding chemically changed cholesterol products not normally found in food produces artery disease in test animals.

Even before this latest pricking of the cholesterol-as-cause-of-artery-disease bubble, another significant finding emerged. Because it turned out that not all strains of rabbits react to cholesterol feeding as did those used by Anitschkow, a group of investigators headed by Dr. K.B. Turner looked into the matter in 1938. They found that if those rabbits susceptible to cholesterol-feeding were given therapeutic doses of thyroid, the blood cholesterol levels were lowered and atherosclerosis did not develop. On the other hand, if they removed the thyroids from rabbits resistant to cholesterol-feeding, they promptly developed high blood levels of cholesterol and atherosclerosis. It seemed that thyroid deficiency was more important for the development of atherosclerosis in rabbits than was the presence of excess cholesterol.

And, fittingly enough, still later, in 1964, from an investigator, L.V. Malysheva, in Russia where the cholesterol experiments had started came word that before atherosclerosis developed in cholesterol-fed rabbits, the metabolism of these animals fell to levels as low as those seen in rabbits with thyroid glands removed.

The Circumstantial Web

Meanwhile, however, shortly after Anitschkow's work had called attention to cholesterol, a web of circumstantial evidence began to be built against the substance. In 1916, a Dutch physician, Dr. C.D. DeLangen, working in Java, reported that the people of that country had lower blood cholesterol levels than those found in Holland and their incidence of atherosclerosis was lower. And, it was noted, the diet in Java was lower in cholesterol.

Soon, other reports began to indicate that countries with diets high in vegetables but low in animal products generally had populations with lower cholesterol levels and fewer heart attacks than meat-eating nations. And this was evidence which Dr. White, among many others, held to be highly significant.

World War II was, for proponents of the cholesterol theory, an unsought-for experiment par excellence. Millions of people were forced to change their eating habits during the war, especially in Europe. Cholesterol-containing foods were in short supply or not available at all and the incidence of heart attacks fell remarkably. As soon as the war was over and cholesterol-rich foods returned, heart attacks again climbed and went up to even greater heights.

It seemed to some cholesterol-theory enthusiasts that there could not possibly be any other reason than the change in diet for the fluctuations in the incidence of heart attacks. Yet, as pointed out earlier in this chapter, there was another reason: the fluctuations in infectious disease, including tuberculosis, and the effects of these fluctuations on the heart attack rate.

Cholesterol-theory enthusiasts were intrigued by the rarity of heart attacks in underdeveloped countries where cholesterol intake was low. And yet these reports could be misleading if not very carefully analyzed.

Right at the end of World War II, in 1945, a report was

published on 3,000 consecutive autopsies among the
Bantu of South Africa during the years 1924 to 1938.
Only six cases of heart attacks were found. It sounded
like a remarkably low incidence.

But one-fourth of all the deaths were due to tuberculosis, which kills young adults. Many other deaths were
due to other infectious diseases which also kill the young.
Among the 3,000 people autopsied, only 352 had reached
age fifty. Six heart attacks in a population of 352 reaching
an age level when they are most likely candidates are far
different from 6 in 3,000. It seems more likely that the
killing off of people susceptible to infectious diseases
rather than low cholesterol diet was responsible for the
low incidence of heart attacks.

Interestingly, too, the autopsies at Graz in 1930, about
the same time as the Bantu study, showed that deaths
from tuberculosis in Graz were also high, accounting for
17 percent of the total. In Graz, there were 13 heart
attacks in 769 people over the age of fifty who came to
autopsy. Thus, the incidence of heart attacks for the
Bantu and for the people of Graz was the same, yet the
Bantu ate little cholesterol while the Austrians had a
relatively high intake.

The World Health Organization reported a sharp
drop in tuberculosis among black South Africans during
the 1950s. Not surprisingly, with the reduction in tuberculosis incidence, the heart attack incidence has been
increasing.

In 1954, a report of 523 autopsies among the Bantu
found tuberculosis accounting for 12 percent of deaths,
about half the former rate. But the heart attack rate had
increased fourfold and every one of the 523 patients
autopsied showed some early atherosclerosis.

In 1960, it became apparent that younger patients with heart attacks were appearing among the Bantu as deaths from infections were reduced. In a period of six months in one medical ward, six patients died of heart attacks; one was only twenty-two years of age, two were forty, one forty-eight, one fifty-eight, and one sixty-five.

The Japanese experience is of interest. At one point, it seemed to cholesterol-theory proponents that Japan provided evidence in favor of the value of a low cholesterol diet in preventing heart attacks. In 1956, when an analysis was made of 10,000 autopsies carried out in Japan over a period of forty years, it was estimated that the heart attack rate was only one-tenth that of the United States. It is significant that the World Health Organization figures at the time of the autopsy analysis indicated that the death rate from tuberculosis in Japan was twelve times that in the United States. And in recent years, as the death rate from tuberculosis and other infectious diseases in Japan has been lowered markedly, the incidence of heart attacks has risen markedly.

A Personal Awakening

My personal interest in heart attacks was not aroused until 1950 when a friend, a fifty-nine-year-old navy retiree, developed severe chest pain while traveling by car 60 miles from home. How he ever managed to drive home and survive is still a mystery. An electrocardiogram showed that he had suffered a severe heart attack. Three days later, he suffered another attack.

He had been in seeming good health all his life, right up to the first heart attack. He had not been a patient of mine and in fact rarely had seen any physician before. When I took a thorough medical history, however, it became apparent that he had had symptoms for several years of hypothyroidism for which he had sought no medical advice.

He came through the two heart attacks and after resting for more than a month went back to his normal activities. Two years later, he was started on thyroid therapy and for seven years led an active, vigorous life, even coming out of retirement to take on a challenging executive job. He became negligent about his thyroid medication and had been off thyroid for four months when he died of another heart attack at the age of sixty-eight.

This was the first heart attack case in my practice. For many years I had been carefully screening new patients for evidence of thyroid deficiency and had been combating their susceptibility to infections, their menstrual irregularities, their fatigue and depression, and other symptoms associated with deficiency by means of thyroid therapy. There hadn't been any heart attacks. Was this pure coincidence? Or did it have significance?

This was at a time when the rapidly rising incidence of coronary artery disease and heart attacks was causing concern. By 1950, it was obvious that many cases of heart attacks were accompanied by high blood cholesterol levels. To most investigators, this suggested that the elevated cholesterol levels were causing the attacks, but to me they signaled possible thyroid deficiency. The thyroidectomized baby rabbits I had used in my physiology course had had high cholesterol levels. I recalled, too, the work of Dr. Hurxthal at the Lahey Clinic demonstrating in human patients that the thyroid controls the cholesterol level.

Certainly, the role of thyroid deficiency in heart disease ought to be studied. Since my practice was devoted increasingly to patients with thyroid deficiency and new ones with deficiency were constantly appearing, it would be possible over a period of years to observe the influence of thyroid therapy on the incidence of heart attacks.

The Plan

Beginning in 1950, my pretreatment examinations for new patients were broadened to include a chest X-ray for heart size, an electrocardiogram, and blood studies including checks for cholesterol levels. In order to run a valid scientific study, only one factor at a time must be changed if the influence of that factor is to be pinpointed. Hence, patients were not asked to change any of their routine habits—to stop smoking, exercise more, try to avoid stress, or adopt a low-fat, low-cholesterol diet.

In fact, overweight patients were encouraged to eat an abundance fat meat, bacon and eggs for breakfast, cheese, extra butter or oleo on their vegetables, and salads with oil in the dressings. This was in keeping with a reducing diet which I have always found effective and will be suggested later in the chapter on obesity.

There was no worry that such a diet would raise blood cholesterol levels since thyroid was to be used to keep the level within normal range. And in 95 percent of the patients who used that diet, the blood cholesterol level did stay within normal range. Even in the patients in whom the level did not come down to normal and in a very few in whom it remained at fairly high levels of 300 or more, the diet was continued along with thyroid therapy and in not one case has a heart attack occurred.

The Protective Effect

A total of 1,569 patients were in the study. Some were in it for the full twenty years; some for lesser amounts of time, coming into it at various points as it progressed. But no patient was included in analysis of the results unless he or she had been participating for at least two years.

At the end of the twenty years, only four heart attacks had occurred. These were in men. The youngest was fifty-six; his father had died with the same disease at the age of fifty-two. The oldest was sixty-one, a man who gave little thought to his health, often trying to get by on two or three hours' sleep a night and pushing himself beyond his endurance. In these four cases, the thyroid dosage was only two grains a day; viewed in retrospect, the dosage may have been inadequate. Of the 1,569 patients observed for a total of 8,824 patient-years, 844 were women; there were no heart attacks among them.

Ideally, in carrying out a scientific study, there should be a control group. In addition to those receiving treatment, there should be others not receiving treatment and serving for comparison. But in private practice, this is not easily achieved. To have denied appropriate therapy to any of these patients coming to me for help would have constituted malpractice.

Fortunately, the government's famed Framingham

study provided a good basis for comparison. The study—officially termed the Heart Disease Epidemiology Study—was started in 1949 by the National Heart Institute. Ever since, it has been following closely more than 5,000 men and women in the Massachusetts community of Framingham, near Boston. Its major purpose has been to determine which of these people, healthy to begin with, would develop evidence of coronary heart disease and to try to clarify the factors that led to the disease.

Detailed observations were made on each person in the study to determine life habits, familial traits, environmental characteristics, and other factors that might conceivably turn out to be related to the development of heart disease.

Of the people participating in the Framingham study, some eight hundred have died, many of them from heart attacks. The study has underscored facts about various factors in heart attacks: that the disease is more frequent in men, that a family history of the disease increases the risk, that a high blood cholesterol level and/or high blood pressure is a predisposing factor, and that the frequency of heart attacks increases with age.

Those participating in the Framingham study did not receive thyroid therapy. And by grouping thyroid-treated patients into the same classifications used in the Framingham study, comparisons can be made of the incidence of heart disease in the thyroid-treated and those not receiving thyroid therapy.

And such comparisons are shown in Table 1 which breaks down the 1,569 thyroid-treated patients and groups them in the six classifications used in the

Table 1

Sex	Classification	Number of patients treated	Patient years	Expected coronary cases according to Framingham	Actual coronary cases observed
F	Age 30-59	490	2,705	7.6	0
F	High-risk (with high cholesterol levels or high blood pressure or both)	172	1,086	7.3	0
F	Age over 60	182	955	7.8	0
M	Age 30-59	382	2,192	12.8	1
M	High-risk (with high cholesterol levels or high blood pressure, or both)	186	1,070	18.5	2
M	Age over 60	157	816	18.0	1
	TOTALS	1,569	8,824	72.0	4

Framingham study. The table indicates the number of patients in each group and the patient-years of thyroid treatment and also indicates the number of coronary disease cases to be expected in each group according to the experience in Framingham and the number that actually occurred in each group.

Thus, based on the Framingham experience, there should have been twenty-two heart attacks among the women and fifty among the men, or a total of seventy-two, among the 1,569 thyroid treated patients. There were only 4.

The results indicate that 94 percent of those who, without thyroid therapy, should have been candidates for heart attacks during the study were protected from them by thyroid therapy.

On a statistical basis, smoking has been accused of making a major contribution to heart attacks. In spite of propaganda to the contrary and in spite of the fact that I myself quit smoking in 1920 for financial reasons, patients in the study were told that evidence that smoking was a significant factor was inconclusive and no one was asked to stop smoking. Many of the women were cigarette smokers and 62 percent of the men were.

Although there is no doubt that statistics indicate that smokers have more heart attacks, the case is far from being open and shut. The smoker is often a tired person and smoking elevates the blood sugar a little and may provide a temporary lift. He may well be hypothyroid and that condition would make him more susceptible to atherosclerosis whether he smoked or not. It is not safe to compare his liability to atherosclerosis with that of the nonsmoker unless all other factors are ruled out. This has not been done.

Lack of adequate exercise is another debatable factor alleged to be operating in the rise in heart attack incidence. In the thyroid-treated patients, no extra exercise was advised. They continued to do what they had done before. I have always believed that if an individual has enough energy to enjoy exercise, he can do it for pleasure and he will quit when he is tired. On the other hand, if he is encouraged "to protect his health by exercise," there is a danger that he may overexert.

We still must search for what it is that makes the male sex on the whole more prone to infectious diseases and to heart attacks than women. There is little if any difference in the resistance of the sexes until the time of puberty. It is about that time that the male begins to expend more energy than the female. At that point, he engages more and more in vigorous competitive sports, often gets part-time jobs, and not infrequently may devote considerable attention to exercises to build up his muscle mass.

Is the male sacrificing some resistance for the sake of his strength? It is impossible to say at the present, but it is a fact that early success in treating tuberculosis didn't involve setting the patient to jogging but rather putting him to bed. At the moment, we simply do not have any accurate data to indicate beyond question that longevity is increased by strenuous exercise.

The Dropouts

Evidence of the importance of thyroid therapy comes not only from the results in the 1,569 patients receiving such treatment in the study but also from the results in patients who dropped out for various reasons. Some moved to other areas and their new physicians declined to continue the treatment. Some did not care to take a pill every day after their symptoms of thyroid deficiency disappeared.

At least thirty fatal heart attacks are known to have occurred among those who stopped thyroid treatment. A high proportion of the victims were young. Two were under the age of thirty, one was between thirty and forty, two were between forty and fifty, and eight were between fifty and sixty. These were all premature attacks, indicating an increased susceptibility to atherosclerosis in younger people with thyroid deficiency. Each of these patients had been found thyroid deficient several years before at which time there was no evidence of heart disease.

The youngest dropout to die was a twenty-four-year-old man who was first seen with a thyroid deficiency at the age of seventeen and became free of symptoms on thyroid therapy. He went away to college soon afterward and stopped treatment since he felt that his problems were solved. Without warning, he collapsed a month after graduating from college. I arrived within ten minutes after his mother called, but he was dead. Autopsy revealed that both major coronary arteries were almost completely closed off by atherosclerosis. His mother then confessed that heart attacks had been frequent among her relatives but she had not wanted to let her son know about this for fear it would worry him. Yet, an awareness of his increased susceptibility might have prompted him to keep on with his thyroid treatment which might well have left him a healthy man instead of a death statistic.

The Case Studies

If I had ever thought that I deserved any congratulations for discovering the value of thyroid therapy as an effective prophylaxis against heart attacks, I would have been in for a rude awakening.

Well before the end of the twenty-year study, it was evident that thyroid treatment was having a marked effect. And, belatedly, I decided to review the medical literature, including the early literature, on thyroid physiology, to see if there had been any previous indications of a relationship between the thyroid and the heart.

And previous indications there had been, indeed. They had even been there before heart attacks were actually recognized for what they are.

You'll recall the work of Dr. William M. Ord which we discussed to some extent in an earlier chapter. In 1877, Ord performed an autopsy at St. Thomas Hospital in London on a fifty-eight-year-old woman. She had suffered from many symptoms over a four-year period: difficulty in keeping warm, urinary infection, loss of muscular power, backache, and swelling of the skin of her whole body with her face becoming puffy and expressionless.

In performing the autopsy, Ord noticed the presence of a large amount of jellylike mucin which held water and caused swelling all over the body as well as in the skin. Ord's autopsy was thorough. He noticed that the thyroid gland was almost completely destroyed—and he also noticed that the heart was enlarged and that many arteries were diseased, containing deposits of foreign material that narrowed them greatly.

It was apparent at once that something new had been discovered in medicine. Other physicians recognized cases they had not understood. Further study was needed and the Clinical Society of London created one of the earliest "think tanks" on December 14, 1883. Dr. Ord and twelve other leading clinicians and scientists were appointed to make a detailed investigation of thyroid deficiency. This learned group collected cases of myxedema from around the world and sought the observations of all surgeons known to have done thyroidectomies. Sir Victor Horsley, a London physiologist, carried out thyroidectomies in several species of animals and followed the development of myxedema in them.

Five years later the report of a Committee of The Clinical Society of London to Investigate the Subject of MYXEDEMA was published and its 317 pages are worth study in detail by anyone interested in thyroid physiology. Undoubtedly the correspondence of the Committee with Professor Billroth, a distinguished Vienna surgeon who was carrying out total thyroidectomies to prevent suffocation in patients with huge goiters, aroused his interest in the effects of thyroid deficiencies. Routine autopsies in Vienna would have shown the damage to the arteries in those losing their thyroids. And it is no surprise that one of Billroth's students, Dr. von Eiselsberg, as early as 1895, began to thyroidectomize sheep and goats to study the effects on the arteries. He reported finding atherosclerosis developing in the big main artery, the aorta, and also in the coronary arteries feeding the heart. These observations were confirmed by other Viennese investigators who also noted that thyroid administration would prevent the artery damage.

The influence of thyroid deficiency on the artery system became so well-known in Vienna that in his first book on the ductless or endocrine glands, Dr. Wilhelm Falta in 1913 defined myxedema as a condition in which, among other changes, the arteries become prematurely damaged by atherosclerosis.

It is unfortunate that these clear demonstrations of the role of thyroid deficiency in the development of atherosclerosis were forgotten. But heart attacks had not been described then.

In 1918, a German physician, Dr. H. Zondek, focussed attention again on thyroid deficiency and the heart. He had under his care a number of patients bedridden with heart failure which did not respond to digitalis, a drug long used to help such patients. Some of these patients, Zondek noticed, had a myxedematous appearance and when he tried thyroid therapy their response was remarkable. Their enlarged hearts shrank to normal size, their edema disappeared, and they were able to resume normal activities. Zondek coined the term "myxedema heart" for the problem, an unfortunate term since many patients may have heart failure due to thyroid deficiency without developing the facial changes of myxedema. A few of Zondek's patients died before thyroid therapy could be started and autopsies showed marked atherosclerosis, especially of the coronary arteries.

It wasn't long before many physicians were confirming Zondek's findings. Typical was a report by Dr. H.A. Christian, a Rhode Island physician, in 1925. His patients, like Zondek's, responded to thyroid therapy. One of them was a woman who was seventy-three years old when heart failure became evident. She had been treated for thyroid deficiency for twenty-five years and the heart failure developed only when she stopped taking thyroid. When she was put back on two grains of thyroid a day, the heart failure disappeared.

One of Christian's patients died suddenly before thyroid therapy could be started. Again, autopsy revealed that the coronary arteries were narrowed because of atherosclerosis.

And More Needless Confusion

Some American physicians were in a hurry. They were eager for quick results and they started patients on large doses of thyroid. They had been accustomed to saturating the patient in heart failure with sizeable quantities of digitalis, then cutting the medication back for maintenance.

Unfortunately, saturating the patient with thyroid produced too much stimulation of the heart over too short a period; angina pain and heart attack appeared in a few patients. In 1925, a report from physicians at the Peter Bent Brigham Hospital in Boston appeared in *The Journal of the American Medical Association* and pointed out the dangers of overdosage with thyroid. It recommended starting with one grain a day and cautiously raising the dosage. Usually two grains a day were all that was needed to maintain the patient free of heart failure.

It seems likely that thyroid therapy would have taken its rightful place in the treatment and prevention of premature heart disease had it not been for another unfortunate therapeutic error.

In 1938, one physician published a stern warning about the dangers of thyroid therapy in cases of coronary disease. He collected eight deaths from the medical literature and added one of his own, all occurring after thyroid therapy was started. He had started his patient on four grains of thyroid daily in spite of not only the 1925 report but of others since warning that such large starting doses were risky and needless. On the eighth day of overdosage a heart attack occurred.

A review of the eight other cases collected by this physician revealed that in every one of them, the same overdosage pattern applied. The smallest starting dose had been four grains of thyroid and the largest, thirty grains a day. If this were a common practice, it would have been amazing that more deaths were not reported. Such abuse of digitalis therapy would almost invariably have produced death.

Hundreds of lives had been prolonged with judicious use of thyroid therapy yet the 1938 report focused attention on nine deaths not really from thyroid therapy but from physician error.

As a result of that report, a kind of phobia arose against use of thyroid in patients with heart disease. It has been an uphill fight to reorient the medical profession since then, but progress is being made.

Some More Rays of Light

Not all was confusion. Sporadic reports continued to implicate thyroid deficiency in artery degeneration. Only a few can be mentioned here for lack of space.

In New York, at the Bronx Hospital Laboratory, confirming animal studies—this time with lambs—were carried out. In Russia, an investigator working in the same laboratory where earlier cholesterol feeding had produced atherosclerosis in rabbits reported that thyroid administration with the cholesterol feeding prevented artery damage. He went on to suggest that thyroid therapy be used as a prophylaxis against human heart disease.

Dr. T. Leary, the Boston medical examiner, accumulated nine cases of deaths from heart attacks in patients under forty years of age. He not only did thorough autopsy studies showing the clogging deposits in the coronary arteries of these patients but also repeated the cholesterol feeding to rabbits and concluded that deposits were not laid down in the arteries until mucoid degeneration had taken place. He had no idea what caused the mucoid degeneration but he was aware that in some way the thyroid was involved.

In 1951, Dr. William B. Kountz of the Washington University School of Medicine, St. Louis, published a significant report on thyroid function and blood vessel degeneration. He had worked with three groups of patients to see if thyroid therapy was beneficial. The first group consisted of businessmen with an average age of fifty-five years, the second was made up of infirmary outpatients with an average age of sixty-one years, and the third consisted of hospitalized patients with an average age of sixty-seven years. The three groups totaled 288 patients.

All the patients had high blood cholesterol levels and all had low metabolic rates. There was little evidence of atherosclerosis in the youngest age group, moderate damage in the middle group, and far advanced deterioration in the oldest patients.

Over a five-year period, some of the patients in each group received thyroid therapy while others, for comparison, did not. During that time, among the businessmen on thyroid therapy there were no deaths from either heart attacks or strokes, but 15 percent of the other businessmen not receiving thyroid died from either heart attack or stroke. In the second group, death occurred in 3 percent of the thyroid treated and in six times as many, 19 percent, of those not receiving thyroid. Even in the third group, older and with advanced artery deterioration, deaths were one-half as frequent among the thyroid-treated as among those not receiving thyroid.

And More "Comedy of Errors"

In 1954, a group of investigators at the University of California, having become convinced that elevated levels of cholesterol and fats in the blood were a major factor in coronary disease, decided to test the ability of thyroid to reduce these levels below normal. They began with patients in a mental institution who did not have thyroid deficiency. It appeared that about five grains of thyroid were needed.

The error came when the investigators went on to use five grains of thyroid in patients who were not normal, who had not only elevated cholesterol and fats but in many cases coronary heart disease as well. The lesson of thirty years before—that such patients cannot tolerate starting doses of four grains, let alone five—evidently had been overlooked. Angina and heart attacks followed. Once again, thyroid therapy had a black eye because of physician error.

There was too much evidence in the literature implicating thyroid function in atherosclerosis to abandon efforts to try to control the artery disease with thyroid therapy. But instead of using the smaller doses of thyroid that had been found effective in hundreds of cases, there was a hunt to find a synthetic derivative of thyroid hormone which might lower blood cholesterol levels without raising metabolism and causing angina.

When nature produces a compound for use in living organisms, the compound always has the characteristic of rotating polarized light to the left. When the chemist synthesizes a compound in the laboratory, he may obtain equal amounts of two forms of the compound, one rotating polarized light to the left and the other rotating it to the right. Very often, the compound rotating the light to the right—and known as the dextro form—has less physiological activity than the natural or levo form.

Sure enough, when the dextro form of thyroxine, a thyroid hormone, was synthesized, it proved to have only one-tenth to one-twentieth of the metabolic activity of the natural Levo-thyroxine.

Next, attempts to lower blood cholesterol levels with Dextro-thyroxine, or as it is more familiarly known, D-thyroxine, were undertaken. Large doses of the compound were necessary but the cholesterol did fall some.

And now came another error. The dosage of D-thyroxine recommended by the manufacturer for lowering serum cholesterol was four to eight milligrams a day. But while D-thyroxine had less metabolic activity than L-thyroxine and thyroid extract, four to eight milligrams of it a day would have as much metabolic activity as four to eight grains of thyroid extract a day.

The medical profession was assured by salesmen, by brochures, and by advertising in medical journals that with such dosage cholesterol could be lowered effectively and safely.

Some of our leading scientists were misled to the point that D-thyroxine was included with other compounds in a national study carried out at a number of medical centers and aimed at lowering cholesterol levels. The study was double-blind, meaning that neither the patients participating nor the physicians would know who was receiving which compound until the study was over and the secret code was broken. In the study, six milligrams of D-thyroxine were to be used—the equivalent of four and a half grains of dessicated thyroid.

But something went very wrong. Too many patients were dying. The study had to be interrupted and the code broken. It turned out that D-thyroxine was the culprit. It was discarded from the study.

Despite the "comedy of errors"—more appropriately it could be called the tragedy of errors since it has delayed effective use of thyroid therapy for many patients and cost many lives—other investigators have plowed ahead. At least two other serious attempts to use thyroid therapy in proper dosage should be mentioned.

Dr. M. Israel, a New York City clinician, has published several studies in which he has demonstrated repeatedly that thyroid therapy is not only safe but effective in controlling atherosclerosis in patients with demonstrated disease.

In 1971, Dr. James C. Wren reported an extensive five-year study with 347 patients, 173 men and 174 women. He wanted to determine the possible effects of thyroid therapy on the course of atherosclerosis in these patients.

The atherosclerosis was symptomatic in 132 of the patients whose mean age was 64.5 years. Some had experienced a heart attack; some had had a stroke; some suffered from angina pectoris. There were others who were suffering difficulties with leg circulation because of atherosclerosis in the leg arteries. Some had electrocardiographic evidence of atherosclerosis of the coronary arteries.

The 215 patients with asymptomatic atherosclerosis had a mean age of 54.7 years and were considered high risks because of the presence of electrocardiographic abnormalities, high blood pressure, diabetes, or high cholesterol levels.

Only 9 percent of the patients—31 of the total 347 —proved to be hypothyroid by the usual laboratory tests. Nevertheless, all were treated with thyroid and substantial clinical improvement occurred in a significant number of patients in both groups. The mean cholesterol levels fell by 22 percent. Of 41 patients who had angina at the start of the study, 29 reported benefits that included increased exercise tolerance, decreased frequency and severity of attacks, and less need for nitroglycerin.

The great majority of the symptomatic patients, 100 of

the 132, reported benefits from thyroid treatment in the form of increased sense of well-being, greater alertness, increased ability to be active.

And the death rate was less than was to be expected. Eleven patients died during the study. Their mean age was seventy-five, and ten of the eleven had had a heart attack or other symptomatic episode of atherosclerosis before treatment began. The death rate was less than half—44 percent—of the expected rate based on U.S. Life Tables.

Atherosclerosis has been looked upon as irreversible. But Dr. Wren's results indicate that administration of thyroid may be of benefit in many cases and some degree of modification or prevention of progression of the artery disease appears possible even after heart attacks or other serious events.

My own experience has been the same. Mine has been a limited experience—fortunately—because so very few of my patients who have been found hypothyroid and have been placed on thyroid therapy have had heart attacks or other serious events. But I have seen a small number of patients who have sought help after a heart attack. It has been my practice to treat a patient with a heart attack in the customary manner for sixty days—with bed rest and gradual resumption of activity. After the sixty-day period, I begin administering thyroid therapy in a dose of only one-half grain daily. The basal temperature is checked periodically and if the temperature is in the normal range, the dosage is maintained as is. If the basal temperature is still below normal, the dosage may be increased by one-quarter grain increments at two- or three-month intervals as needed. The maximum dosage in patients having had a heart attack is two grains a day.

Such treatment has proved safe and the survival rate has been excellent. Most patients have resumed their previous work and have been able to lead normal lives.

A Rational Approach

Thyroid deficiency can produce many changes in the body which encourage heart attacks. One of the most important is the deposition in abnormal amounts of mucopolysaccharides in the tissues as we have seen earlier, and these are the compounds known to accumulate early in any injury or inflammation and in atherosclerosis.

But there are other changes. In some cases, blood pressure is elevated and thyroid therapy lowers the pressure in most of these, taking extra work off the heart. Swiss investigators many years ago demonstrated that in hypothyroidism, blood clotting is accelerated and heart attacks often occur when a clot blocks completely a narrowed, atherosclerotic artery. With thyroid therapy, blood clotting activity returns to normal.

Another important factor is fatigue. If overexertion can trigger a heart attack, what constitutes overexertion depends upon the condition of the individual. For a chronically tired person, an extra energy expenditure that could be taken in stride by a vigorous person may constitute overexertion. Thyroid deficiency is a common cause of undue fatigue.

A rational approach to the prevention of heart attacks

calls for the recognition of thyroid deficiency—better late than never but preferably as early as possible—and its proper treatment for the rest of life.

Nor is it difficult to recognize thyroid deficiency. Laboratory tests as yet are not precise enough to do so in every case. Symptoms alone, however, can provide clues—and they can be any of the symptoms discussed in earlier chapters since the thyroid affects every cell in the body.

And the basal temperature test has proved to be satisfactory for many years in confirming a suspicion that thyroid deficiency is present and in serving as a guide to its proper correction.

12

Arthritis

OUR ANCESTORS CALLED IT RHEUMATISM but the modern physician calls it arthritis. There has been no change in the disease except the price has gone up with the new name. Instead of an office call fee of $3 for rheumatism, it is now many times that for arthritis.

Although the incidence of arthritis is not much different from that of hypertension, the amount of suffering is another matter. Blood pressure may be elevated for years without symptoms but arthritis may begin with debilitating pain even in childhood which may persist into advanced years. There is an old saying that arthritis never kills; it just keeps its victims miserable.

Is there a connection between arthritis and the thyroid? Often there is. I've seen it in hundreds of patients with rheumatic complaints and low thyroid function whose bone, joint, and muscle troubles were relieved when their thyroid function was corrected.

And I have not been alone in seeing this although there has been a vast amount of confusion about the connection. As far back as 1914, in his lectures in New York, Dr. E. Hertoghe, a distinguished Belgian clinician and member of the Royal Academy of Medicine, was pointing out that many patients with rheumatic complaints were improved by thyroid therapy. Among his patients was "an ecclesiastic [who] complained of the stiffness of his knees which rendered ritual genuflection very difficult but which ultimately disappeared." And Hertoghe urged his medical audiences to "think of a possible deficiency of the thyroid secretion" whenever they encountered patients with any of a long list of problems, not least of which are "rheumatoid changes in the muscles, ligaments, or aponeuroses [tendons] ."

Other similar reports followed. Yet they seem to have gotten lost in the shuffle. By 1966, one of the popular medical textbooks on arthritis devoted less than a page to the thyroid gland and arthritis, and dismissed the connection thus: "There is no overt clinical relationship between hyper- or hypothyroidism and the rheumatic states."

But the connection refuses to stay entirely lost. Only four years later, in 1970, a world-renowned British rheumatologist was pointing out that hypothyroidism is a possibility in patients with rheumatic pains. In his report, Dr. D.N. Golding, Consultant in Rheumatology at Princess Alexandra Hospital and Harlow Group of Hospitals in Herts and Essex, England, told of a series of patients with generalized muscle and joint pains, muscle stiffness, and cramps. Some had muscle stiffness that was particularly acute in the morning. Some also had nightly calf muscle cramps.

Fortunately, hypothyroidism was suspected because some of the patients also had such symptoms as lethargy, cold sensitivity, and weight gain. Thyroid administration, Dr. Golding reported, alleviated all the symptoms within a few weeks or, occasionally, months.

Certainly, hypothyroidism cannot be considered to be invariably *the* cause of arthritic conditions. In my practice, I have seen many children and adults respond to thyroid therapy alone. But others have not. More recently, many of these others who had failed to respond to thyroid therapy alone have responded when thyroid has been combined with prednisone, a cortisonelike compound, used in extremely small doses, far below the amounts ever employed before successfully in arthritic conditions and without any of the undesirable effects associated with the larger amounts.

Why Does It Happen?

In 1973, when *The Journal of the American Medical Association* published a *Primer on the Rheumatic Diseases* to keep practicing physicians up to date, sixty-seven different types were discussed. Although dictionaries define rheumatic diseases as affecting the bones, joints, and muscles, other systems may be involved as well, even the blood vessels.

Rheumatic diseases sometimes may arise as a side effect of tuberculosis, syphilis, gonorrhea, and viral diseases such as measles and influenza. But these are relatively uncommon and much about what causes the more common rheumatic diseases which are among the chief causes of chronic disability in the United States has been shrouded in mystery.

Yet there was a clue in the very first case of myxedema described by Dr. Ord in England in 1877, to which we have referred previously. Rheumatism was very much a part of the fifty-four-year-old woman's troubles. Her hands were swollen, her fingers thickened and clumsy, and the range of motion limited. All of her skin and her connective tissues as well were swollen, but the swelling was different than any ever described before. In kidney disease, when fluid is retained in the tissues, the fluid escapes when the surface of the tissues is cut. In this case, however, it did not escape; it was held firmly by something and chemical examination revealed the presence in large amounts of a mucinous substance that had great affinity for water.

When Sir Victor Horsley, an English physiologist, began work at once to try to duplicate myxedema in animals by removing the thyroid gland, he found that soon after the surgery the connective tissues of sheep, donkeys, and other experimental animals had both a high content of the mucinous substance and an abnormal water content.

Later, the mucinous substance was to be found to consist of several compounds now called mucopolysaccharides which have been found to be present in abnormal amounts in many chronic degenerative diseases. In 1950, as we have previously noted, a Danish investigator found an abnormal amount of water-retaining muco-polysaccharides in the skin of patients with hypo-thyroidism. He reported, too, that treatment of such patients with thyroid promptly decreased the skin content of both mucopolysaccharides and water.

In another Danish study five years later, thyroid medication was stopped for six weeks in a group of children who, because of thyroid deficiency, were being maintained on thyroid to promote normal growth and development. In the six-week period, abnormal quantities of mucopolysaccharides collected in the skin; they were promptly reduced to normal levels when thyroid therapy was resumed.

If such deposits of mucopolysaccharides occur in the skin of children with low thyroid function just as they do in thyroidectomized experimental animals, it seems reasonable to believe they occur in other connective tissues of the human body just as they do, too, in the thyroidectomized animals.

The Response in Arthritic Children

Rheumatoid arthritis in children is called Still's disease. It is similar in most respects to the adult type, modified only to the extent that it tends to affect the larger joints and as a result produce changes in growth and development. The outlook is better than in adults. Recovery eventually occurs in 75 to 80 percent of children.

The children with Still's disease whom I have seen in

my practice almost invariably have had histories and physical findings compatible with thyroid deficiency. It appears that other symptoms of hypothyroidism may be present for some time with the arthritis appearing later, particularly at a time of stress.

For example, a twelve-year-old girl I first saw in January 1971 had been in bed for six weeks with swollen, painful joints. She had a long history of repeated colds and sore throats, and had twice had pneumonia, all suggestive of low thyroid function. Both her mother and her maternal grandmother were hypothyroid and there were indications of low thyroid function in her father's side of the family. The child was just beginning to mature, which may have been one stress factor, and another could have been an acute gastrointestinal upset with vomiting which had occurred a few weeks before her arthritis developed.

She was started on a grain of thyroid daily and soon began to improve. She returned to school in a month and has been well since. Although it is not possible to rule out spontaneous recovery, with the thyroid therapy having no real influence on the arthritis, other children have responded similarly, and I believe that the reduction in mucopolysaccharides brought about by therapy with thyroid could explain the prompt improvement.

Adult Arthritics

Who among adults gets arthritis? William Osler, one of America's greatest physicians who helped to establish Johns Hopkins as a major medical school and medical center, was impressed with the histories of infections among his arthritic patients. At that time he felt that infection, when it reached into the joints, could start the arthritic process.

It seems far more likely now that susceptibility to infection is one of the stigma of thyroid deficiency and it is the deficiency which, by predisposing to high levels of mucopolysaccharides, can be an important factor in allowing arthritis to develop.

Actually, many arthritic patients I have seen not only have a history of infections, easy fatigability, and other indications of possible low thyroid function but for many years they have experienced minor joint aches and pains for which they did not seek medical help until their discomfort became acute.

When asked to do so, they usually are able to recall that for five, ten, fifteen, and even twenty years, they experienced transient episodes of joint pain, especially in winter months but rarely in summer. There is a logical explanation for this.

During the winter months, less blood circulates to the extremities and more circulates within the trunk of the body in order to conserve heat. More food also is burned to produce heat and this calls for more thyroid. In the individual with mild hypothyroidism or even borderline thyroid production, thyroid deficiency becomes more pronounced. At that time, mucopolysaccharides may be increased anywhere in the body, including the joints, and the swelling, as more fluid is bound and held, can give rise to pain.

On the other hand, in summer, the demand for thyroid for heat production is far less and circulation to the hands and feet increases for cooling purposes. This would favor resorption of the mucopolysaccharides and reduction in swelling and pain.

Hundreds of patients complaining of mild periodic rheumatism at their first visit have been relieved of it when their other symptoms of thyroid deficiency have been relieved by treatment. And progressive arthritis has been rare among thyroid-treated patients over many years.

The Test Confusion Again

If hypothyroidism is a factor in the development of arthritis, quite reasonably physicians expect that they should be able to demonstrate the concurrence of the two. Here again, as in so many other areas, standard tests have often produced confusion, failing to reveal the hypothyroidism.

A particularly interesting study was made many years ago by Dr. Loring T. Swain, a Boston clinician. He investigated the basal metabolic rate in 312 patients with arthritis. The results seemed to be a puzzle. It didn't matter what the type of arthritis was, some patients with it had a high basal metabolic rate while others had a low rate.

Yet, it's readily apparent now what could have been wrong. To get a reliable basal metabolic rate, the patient must be relaxed, otherwise the rate will be elevated and may even indicate hyperthyroidism despite an actual low thyroid function. Many of these patients must have been in pain at the time of the test and to relax in the presence of pain is quite a feat.

Moreover, many arthritics often tend to run a low-grade fever, sometimes from infection and sometimes because of muscle tension. The basal metabolic rate goes up 10 percent for each degree of above-normal temperature. Obviously, a valid metabolic rate couldn't be obtained in such patients.

Despite the puzzling results he obtained, Dr. Swain went on anyhow to try thyroid therapy in sixty-seven patients. A curious fact that emerged with retesting after some time on thyroid therapy, was that while those in whom the metabolic rate had been originally low showed an elevation, others in whom the rate had been originally high showed a decrease. Dr. Swain interpreted this to mean that those patients in whom the rate came down were under less tension while on thyroid. It is also possible that the lowered rate was associated with fewer episodes of respiratory infection while on thyroid and thus less fever.

Significantly, however, Dr. Swain in treating the sixty-seven patients with thyroid made no attempt to determine the correct dose, simply giving as much as a patient tolerated without undesirable effects. Despite this poor method of administration, the thyroid-treated patients showed improvement in their arthritic symptoms, and in their vitality and feelings of well-being.

Cortisone and Other Corticosteriod Drugs

In 1949, cortisone, a hormone of the adrenal gland, made its appearance and for a time it seemed that arthritis had been conquered. Within a day or two after the powerful compound was administered, pain was relieved, swelling subsided, and normal movement of joints was possible.

Unfortunately, prolonged administration of cortisone could produce bone brittleness, weight gain, ulcer formation, skin eruptions, fluid retention, "moon-shaped" face, depression, and other serious side effects. The "cure" was worse than the disease for many patients and, of course, there was no cure. When cortisone treatment was stopped, there was often a severe rebound phenomenon, and patients could be even worse off than before.

Chemists then went to work to modify the compound, altering its structure and seeking to produce a derivative that would be effective in arthritis and would have fewer serious side effects. And they did turn up new cortisone-related compounds that were an improvement but still hardly solved the problem of arthritis.

The corticosteroids—cortisone and the related compounds—suppressed inflammation. That was well known. What those using the compounds failed to appreciate, however, was the effect of the corticosteroids on thyroid function.

Actually, very quickly after cortisone came into use, just a year later in fact, an extensive study carried out at Harvard showed that corticosteroids have some calorigenic action; that is, they raise the metabolism a little and do so independently of the thyroid. But, of far greater significance, they depress thyroid function.

Here was a clue to why cortisone could be so effective at first but then cause serious side effects and even aggravation of the arthritis. Let us assume for the moment that arthritis is related to hypothyroidism. Cortisone, being anti-inflammatory, could, in the process of suppressing the inflammatory reaction in arthritis, relieve some of the pain. But, after a time, with thyroid function further suppressed by the drug, additional deposits of muco-polysaccharides would appear in the joints—and elsewhere in the body as well—and the arthritis would be worse and side effects would appear.

In the very same study at Harvard, another important fact was turned up. Some patients with low thyroid function failed to respond to cortisone; only when they also received thyroid did their arthritis respond at all to the cortisone.

The study should have suggested the possible value of combining thyroid and corticosteroid for treatment. But apparently the significance of the findings wasn't realized.

The Combination

I first tried combining thyroid therapy and a corticosteroid in 1970. The patient was a middle-aged automobile mechanic who first consulted me in 1967. He had had a partial thyroidectomy seven years before and had been in poor health ever since. Among his complaints were fatigability, palpitations, and some recurrent rheumatism in the wrist and hands.

At the time he was taking medication to further suppress his thyroid function because it was felt it was again hyperactive despite the earlier partial removal of the gland.

I found instead that his thyroid function was low as

indicated by the basal temperature test and by an elevated blood cholesterol level of 307. With thyroid therapy, he showed marked improvement and for three years did very well. Then the arthritis became troublesome. There were more frequent episodes of pain and swelling and now the elbows as well as wrists and hands were affected. Aspirin and other drugs commonly used for arthritis did not help at all.

When he appeared one day with both wrists swollen and fingers so stiff that he could not move them, it was obvious that if such attacks went on, he could no longer work as a mechanic and perhaps at anything else. Reluctantly and rather desperately, I gave him a supply of twenty-one tablets of prednisone, one of the least dangerous of corticosteroids, with the instruction to take one after each meal and return in a week.

When he returned, he was in high spirits, free of pain and swelling, and able to move all joints readily. He was sure he was cured but I warned him to wait a few days before exulting. Soon the pain and swelling returned. This time I gave him more prednisone with instructions to take one tablet after each meal for a few days, then cut the dose to one tablet daily. And the one tablet daily, combined with the thyroid, worked. For four years at this writing, he has continued on the one tablet of prednisone a day combined with thyroid and has been free of pain, fully able to work, and free of any side effects from the corticosteroid.

In the last four years, more than two hundred patients have benefited from the combination treatment. They have ranged from an eighty-six-year-old farmer who had been unable to drive his tractor and use the clutch because of severe knee arthritis to a twenty-three-year-old woman whose first pregnancy precipitated crippling rheumatoid arthritis.

The young mother had been found to be hypothyroid at the age of fourteen, at which point she had a simple goiter and was experiencing menstrual difficulties and other symptoms of hypothyroidism. She did well on a grain of thyroid daily. I didn't see her for more than five years during which she continued on the same dose of thyroid—and she continued on the one grain during her pregnancy.

Soon after her delivery, all her joints became stiff and painful and she could walk only with great pain and difficulty. When I saw her again then, I gradually increased the dosage of thyroid to four grains daily, but only when I added a small dose of prednisone did she become entirely free of pain, swelling, and limited motion, and in fact is now able to ski again. I can't help wondering if proper control of her thyroid deficiency during her pregnancy might not have avoided the arthritis.

Another patient, a thirty-seven-year-old man, was first seen in August 1967. His arthritis had begun in high school and he had been given prednisone from the beginning but was afraid to use it because his father, a severe arthritic, had died of complications from overdosage of cortisone.

When I saw him, he was taking aspirin and a potent noncorticosteroid anti-inflammatory drug, oxyphenbutazone, but was in pain. He was hypothyroid and had other symptoms of low thyroid function, and after three months on two grains of thyroid daily, the other symptoms had disappeared and his arthritic pain had decreased so that he experienced only occasional discomfort in one wrist.

For two years, he did well, but then his arthritis flared. His discomfort was so severe that, unknown to me, he made a trip to Mexico for treatment with a secret wonder drug. For a brief time, it did, indeed, seem to work wonders for him but shortly after his return home he was horrified to learn that the "secret wonder drug" was cortisone in large dosage and he stopped taking it.

For the past two years, he has been maintained on four grains of thyroid and one five-milligram tablet of prednisone morning and evening. During the summer months he is entirely free of pain, but during the winter he may have an occasional episode of minor pain just prior to a change in the weather. He lives in Wyoming where the weather can be extreme in winter. He has been free of any complications from the prednisone. The answer to the problem of undesirable effects seems to be to determine the proper dosage of thyroid by the basal temperature test and then to use the minimum dosage of prednisone to avoid the thyroid-depressing effects that may come with larger dosage.

I should add here that I have seen six other patients who made the trip to Mexico for treatment of arthritis. They saw physicians who spent less than ten minutes with them, charged only modestly for their time, but gave them prescriptions for secret drugs that could be filled only at one pharmacy in the Mexican town at a cost of more than $150 for a six-month supply after which they were to return for another interview with the physicians and another prescription. What they received, as chemical analysis showed, was cortisone in huge dosage. All six were benefited at first, but five were soon worse off than before. All have been placed on thyroid and prednisone and although none is cured, all have shown marked improvement.

One of my patients, a woman in her seventies, first came to see me in 1957 with minor arthritis which was readily controlled with an aspirinlike compound, sodium salicylate. Four years later she had an attack of bursitis in her right shoulder and shortly thereafter her right knee became swollen and painful. At that time, I found her to be hypothyroid and she was started on one grain a day of thyroid with considerable relief. Later the dosage was raised to two grains a day and that was continued for fourteen years.

For much of the time, she did well, but then she began to have occasional flareups of knee pain and swelling. The flareups were relieved promptly by one of the old treatments for arthritis that has been all but abandoned: an intravenous injection of sodium salicylate, sodium iodide, and colchicine. Within two hours after the injection, she would experience relief which would last for weeks and sometimes months.

For the last four years, she has been on thyroid and prednisone and remains free of pain without injections. In the beginning, she needed to take only five milligrams of prednisone only once every several days. For the past two years, she has needed five milligrams once a day. She is not cured of arthritis, of course, but at age seventy-two she is free of discomfort, able to get around without restrictions, and free of any undesirable effects.

Gouty Arthritis

A special form of arthritis is that due to gout which is much more common in men than women. In the classic case, the big toe becomes swollen, inflamed, and excruciatingly painful, but any joint may be similarly affected. The swelling, inflammation, and pain are due to deposits of uric acid in the joint, settling there out of the blood. The blood content of uric acid is usually higher than normal and the excretion rate of the uric acid through the kidneys is lower than normal.

Sometimes, uric acid may be deposited in the kidneys causing the formation of stones that may block the excretion of urine. One patient in whom this happened was a forty-two-year-old man who was hypothyroid, had had arthritis in his knees, and responded well to two grains of thyroid daily for five years. When he developed urinary difficulty, he was hospitalized, found to have a high blood uric acid level, and a large stone in a kidney interfering with urinary drainage.

After his recovery from the stone incident, his thyroid dosage was increased to four grains daily. The stone incident occurred sixteen years ago. On thyroid therapy alone, he has had no recurrence of gout and his serum uric acid has been normal.

The uric acid level of the blood is often high in hypothyroid patients although they do not all have gout.

The uric acid level usually falls when thyroid therapy is instituted. But some cases of gouty arthritis require colchicine for relief and colchicine and/or other specific anti-gout drugs to prevent recurrences. Thyroid therapy is not specific for gout but it can be a valuable adjunct to treatment when elevated serum uric acid is associated with hypothyroidism.

13

The Thyroid, Diabetes, and Hypoglycemia

THERE WERE FORTY TWO DIABETIC PATIENTS. They were using insulin or tolbutamide or another oral antidiabetic drug. Because of low basal temperatures, they were placed on thyroid therapy. About two months after the proper dosage of thyroid had been determined, they began to have fewer infections, wounds healed promptly, blood fat levels returned to normal, and they experienced feelings of greater well-being and increased energy. Over a period of many years, the complications of diabetes have been conspicuous by their absence. No gangrene, kidney failure, stroke, blindness, or neuropathies have occurred. Only one patient has suffered a heart attack.

Diabetes, we know today, is an "iceberg" disease. It involves more than sugar in the blood. Indeed, the sugar in the blood is only the tip of the iceberg.

214

Despite the euphoric feelings of half a century ago after the discovery of insulin that diabetes was a disease that no longer would be a problem, it remains a formidable problem. It is no longer so much a problem of controlling the metabolic aspect of the disease, the hyperglycemia, or excess of sugar in the blood, resulting from faulty handling of carbohydrates. Diabetics today aren't so much troubled by and they rarely die now of metabolic crises. But many suffer from the complications of diabetes—from blindness, kidney and nervous disease, skin infections and, above all, degenerative changes in the heart and blood vessels. They have twice the rate of coronary heart disease as do nondiabetics. At the world-famed Joslin Clinic in Boston, 46.5 percent of deaths in diabetics have been reported due to atherosclerotic heart disease. And as many as 77 percent of deaths in diabetics are due to blood vessel disease of one type or another.

Thyroid therapy can do much to help many diabetics, as I think you will see. The complications of diabetes are much like the manifestations of hypothyroidism. Many diabetics do, in fact, have low thyroid function. I am not the first by any means to make that observation and there have been findings by others as well that suggest that the complications of diabetes, particularly the atherosclerotic complications, are not due to the disturbance in carbohydrate metabolism but to something else. And that something else could well be hypothyroidism. Which would mean that thyroid therapy should help. And, in my experience, it does help. I believe, too, that thyroid therapy for people with low thyroid function who have not yet developed diabetes may do much to prevent appearance of the disease.

The Sugar Problem

Normally, all the carbohydrate foods we eat—the sugars and starches—are converted in the intestinal tract and in the liver to glucose, a simple sugar also called dextrose. About 60 percent of the protein food we eat is also convertible to glucose. Glucose goes by way of the blood to all body tissues where it is used to produce the energy needed for functioning.

Normally, the sugar level in the blood is regulated precisely. Between meals, the level lies between 80 and 100 milligrams of glucose for every 100 milliliters of blood. When a meal is being absorbed, the blood sugar rises but usually does not exceed 160 milligrams. The hormone insulin lowers the sugar level by promoting the rapid entry of glucose into most cells where it is needed.

Insulin is produced by certain cells, called beta cells, in the islets of Langerhans in the pancreas. Normally, when blood sugar goes up for any reason, the rise stimulates the beta cells to secrete a small amount of insulin which then regulates the blood sugar level.

If the beta cells are disturbed and unable to quickly secrete an adequate amount of insulin, the blood sugar level will rise. If it goes above 180 or 200 milligrams, the kidney will excrete the extra sugar.

Diabetes comes from a Greek word meaning to run through. And in diabetes glucose does run through the body to be excreted in the urine. In doing so, it increases the demand for water and may produce great thirst along with increased urination. Other symptoms may include loss of weight, sometimes with increased appetite and excessive food intake; weakness; itching of genitals and rectum; decreased resistance to infections such as boils and carbuncles and to general infections such as tuberculosis.

At the beginning of this century, the diagnosis of diabetes in a young child was a notice of premature death. Its diagnosis in an adult man or woman meant a complete change in the way of living and greatly reduced expectation of life.

And then, in 1922, two Canadian researchers, Frederick Grant Banting and Charles Herbert Best, isolated insulin and used it to treat diabetic patients. What the two men had discovered in a Toronto laboratory appeared for a time to be a "cure" for the disease.

But it was soon recognized that there were some cases of diabetes which do not respond to insulin. It became apparent that there were two different types of diabetes. One, the juvenile type, affects children, adolescents, and young adults and involves a definite inadequacy of insulin secretion. The other, maturity-onset, tends to occur in middle life; in this type, insulin production may be adequate, but for reasons still not clear the body does not properly respond to the insulin.

Currently, several drugs that can be taken by mouth— including tolbutamide, chlorpropamide, acetohexamide, tolazamide, and phenformin—can be used for maturity-onset diabetes.

Diet, too, is used. The diabetic diet is a measured but normal diet except that the more rapidly absorbed carbohydrates and foods containing them in large amounts must be eaten sparingly. Carbohydrate in the form of starches such as rice and potatoes is preferable to free sugar or high-sugar fruits.

Today, the metabolic aspect of diabetes—the level of sugar in the blood—can be controlled effectively. The complications of diabetes are another matter. They have always been.

The Complications Problem

The most important area of our ignorance about diabetes, as a World Health Organization report noted recently, is the relation of the disorder to various disturbances of the heart and of blood vessels throughout the body. "We must uncover the causes of the more rapid and more extensive arteriosclerosis of the diabetic population, and we must be able to understand the causes of the blood vessel changes in the eyes and kidneys of some diabetics before we can devise effective prevention and treatment," the report emphasized.

Just eight years after the discovery of insulin, it was apparent that the problem of diabetic complications had not been solved and much remained to be done. In 1930, Dr. Elliot P. Joslin, a Boston clinician who devoted his life to diabetes and today is commemorated by the Joslin Clinic, traced progress in the treatment of diabetes in a paper in *The Annals of Internal Medicine*.

In the last century more than half of the diabetics had died of tuberculosis since they were highly susceptible to infections. At that time, the average diabetic patient survived only 4.7 years after his diabetes was diagnosed. As improvements were made in the treatment of tuberculolis, more diabetics began to die of coma. Although they lived about a year longer as the result of surviving tuberculosis, the accumulation of ketone bodies from the burning of fats, which they had to use as the major source of their energy, led to acidosis and death.

Insulin solved this problem because now the diabetic could use sugar and the ketone bodies were eliminated. But a new monster raised its head—hardening of the arteries or atherosclerosis. By 1930, the average diabetic survived only 8.7 years after the disease was diagnosed, and half of diabetic deaths were due to damage to the arteries.

Dr. Joslin was well ahead of his peers. He knew that if patients developed diabetes before the age of fifty, 45 percent of them would die from atherosclerosis. If they did not develop the diabetes until the age of eighty, all of them would die from hardening of the arteries. Obviously, the arterial damage was occurring long before the diabetes appeared; the diabetes did not cause it but only accelerated it.

Unfortunately, most investigators in the diabetic field took the opposite view, holding that the diabetic state was responsible for the artery disease and the problem was to diagnose the diabetes earlier and all would be well.

They overlooked a significant study made in 1919 by a Munich pathologist, G. Hurxheimer, which included a wealth of information from autopsies. At that time, diabetics were surviving on the average less than five years from the time of diagnosis and tuberculosis was the leading cause of death among them at an early age. But even then, Hurxheimer found, 15 percent of them were dying from atherosclerosis. It appeared that individuals susceptible to tuberculosis are also susceptible to atherosclerosis and if the tuberculosis didn't kill, the atherosclerosis had a chance to. This was true in diabetics as well as in nondiabetics.

Twenty years after Joslin had emphasized the importance of atherosclersosis in the diabetic population, atherosclerosis had become the leading cause of death in the *general* population. Heart attacks had replaced tuberculosis as the leading killer; and strokes, kidney failure, and gangrene of the extremities were very much on the rise in the general population.

These were the complications that were killing diabetics, too. They were complications due to atherosclerosis whether they occurred in the heart, the brain, the kidney, or the extremities. There were also many degenerative changes in the eyes and in the nerves of diabetics due to atherosclerosis and reduced blood supply.

Another Study Overlooked

So busy were diabetes investigators with devising methods of diagnosing the disease earlier with the hope that early treatment would prevent the complications that were killing diabetics even though sugar metabolism was rigidly controlled that another significant study was overlooked.

In 1954, Dr. C. D. Eaton, a Detroit physician, published a report in *The Journal of the Michigan Medical Society* entitled "Co-existence of Hypothyroidism with Diabetes Mellitus." In it he told of experience with hundreds of diabetic patients. First of all, he pointed out what is well known but neglected: Symptoms in both diseases are quite similar with the exception of the disturbance in carbohydrate metabolism that occurs in diabetes. The diabetic patient as well as the hypothyroid patient commonly suffered from one or many of such symptoms as weakness, itching, constipation, somnolence, muscular pains, elevated blood fat levels, susceptibility to infections, poor healing of wounds, premature atherosclerosis, and gangrene.

It was common, Dr. Eaton noted, to control the sugar level in diabetic patients only to have the other symptoms persist. And when he sought to determine the incidence of hypothyroidism in diabetic patients by means of the basal metabolic rate, he found that even though that test is not very sensitive and may miss many cases of low thyroid function, it established that hypothyroidism was frequent in diabetics, more so than in the nondiabetic population.

When he then began administration of thyroid in small, physiological doses to his hypothyroid diabetic patients, he found that the thyroid had no influence on the diabetes. When sugar metabolism was controlled by insulin or diet or other measures, it remained controlled when thyroid was added.

But there were other marked changes in his patients whom he saw in the clinic at Grace Hospital in Detroit and in his private practice. They lost their fatigue, their skin problems, and other symptoms of thyroid deficiency which had not been controlled by the control of the diabetes. Their susceptibility to infections decreased greatly.

Dr. Eaton also noted that there were fewer problems with thromboses, or blood clots, in the arteries, which he correctly interpreted as being due to improved circulation and less pooling and stagnation of blood. And he also noted that, as the result of increased circulation in the extremities, there was less gangrene even in those with arteriosclerosis.

The importance of this last observation alone is hard to overemphasize. Consider, for example, a report in 1971 at an American Medical Association meeting by the Joslin Clinic on the diabetic foot. For the year 1969, the cost of hospital admissions, not including physicians' fees, was more than $1 million for foot lesions in diabetic patients. This was for a single institution. Imagine what the total cost across the country is for this problem which Dr. Eaton found could often be avoided by thyroid therapy. It is hardly any wonder that he concluded his 1954 report with the observation that "Thyroid therapy is particularly effective for diabetic patients."

Along with much of the rest of the medical profession, I, too, completely overlooked the Eaton report. I was searching the medical literature for some support for my own observations (made quite independently) on thyroid function and diabetes when I located the Eaton report by accident while reading in the National Library in Washington some eighteen years later. It is a pleasure to confirm every statement he made and to add some of my own observations. Much time has been lost and many diabetics have gone through needless suffering because Eaton's work was overlooked and no one appears to have taken the trouble to confirm or deny this simple approach to the thorny problem of diabetic complications.

Can It Harm?

My interest in diabetes arose while I was still teaching physiology. There had been a report that the diabetes which occurred in dogs after removal of the pancreas would improve when the pituitary gland was also removed. Dr. James Regan and I were the first to confirm this experimental work which had originated in South America. But we also found that other changes after removal of the pituitary—such as wasting away of the thyroid, the adrenals, and the sex glands—were worse than the symptoms of diabetes. And this approach to the treatment of diabetes was dropped.

I did no special research on diabetes after that. In 1950, I began the study on the role of thyroid deficiency in atherosclerosis and heart attacks, following the course of patients placed on thyroid therapy, as discussed in Chapter 11.

While new cases of heart attacks were rare, as we have seen, in the patients receiving thyroid, it was not until 1970 that I realized the possible significance of something else: that some of the treated patients were diabetic and there had been a remarkable absence of complications in them, too.

As a doublecheck to be sure that thyroid therapy could not upset the management of diabetes, a study was carried out at the Norfolk-Nebraska State Hospital with the cooperation of Dr. Robert Osborne. There were forty-two diabetics in the institution. They were divided into two groups. One group was started on one grain of thyroid daily while the other group received a placebo (dummy medication). At the end of a month, the thyroid dosage was raised to two grains daily and at the end of another month the dosage was raised to three grains. After three months, we switched and thyroid was given in exactly the same way to the group which previously had been receiving placebo.

In no patient was any change of diabetic medication necessary whether insulin or oral antidiabetic medication was being used. The diabetes remained as well controlled as before thyroid was used. And, in fact, while thyroid therapy was being used, the diabetes seemed to be under even better control and there were fewer hypoglycemic reactions.

These results, in fact, were in agreement with those of Drs. Campbell Moses and T. S. Danowski of the University of Pittsburgh who had found that although thyroid function tests in diabetics might be normal, as much as three grains of thyroid could be administered daily and would reduce high cholesterol and other blood fat levels.

A Common Dilemma

There appears to be no difference whatever between the atherosclerosis seen in the diabetic and that seen in the nondiabetic. Pathologists have been unable to differentiate between the two. And thyroid therapy is as beneficial in combating the atherosclerosis of the diabetic.

Among the forty-two patients with diabetes who have been in the study extending from 1950 to 1970 and described in Chapter 11, and in other patients with diabetes treated with thyroid since, there has been only a single heart attack. This was in a sixty-seven-year-old woman who had been on thyroid therapy only a short time when the heart attack occurred. It was a minor episode and she recovered quickly.

The absence of progressive loss of vision in this group

of thyroid-treated diabetic patients is most encouraging. Changes in the blood vessels in the eyes of diabetics constitute one of the most common causes of blindness in the United States today. Thyroid therapy appears to be valuable in avoiding this complication.

One of my diabetic patients was sixty-eight years old when she had a heart attack in 1958 at a time when she was not on thyroid. As soon as she had recovered, she was started on thyroid and has taken it ever since. Now at age eighty-four, she is active, takes care of herself, has had no vision impairment and reads her newspaper regularly, and has been entirely free from complications of diabetes since she started on thyroid sixteen years ago.

Another diabetic of long standing is a ninety-three-year-old woman who has been on oral antidiabetic drug and thyroid therapy and whose eyesight remains excellent. She has been free of other complications of diabetes. At age ninety she required gall bladder surgery and her general health was so good that she sailed through it, made a rapid recovery, and was home on the eighth day.

The Oral Antidiabetic Drug Controversy

For several years now there has been a controversy over oral antidiabetic drugs. It began with a serious attempt to determine the best management of diabetics if complications are to be prevented.

Twelve diabetic centers across the country pooled their data in a University Group Diabetes Program. A total of 1,027 diabetics were included in the study. Various types of treatment were used. A preliminary presentation of the data at an American Diabetes Association meeting in June 1970 precipitated the controversy.

Eighty-nine deaths had occurred among the patients, 67 percent of them from atherosclerosis. The atherosclerosis deaths had occurred no matter what the type of treatment for the diabetes, but had been somewhat higher in those receiving an oral antidiabetic drug, tolbutamide, than in those receiving insulin.

It must be remembered that the number of patients involved in the whole study was relatively small. To many physicians, who had used oral antidiabetic drugs for many patients and did not want to abandon their use without overwhelming evidence of harm from them, it seemed that the study had failed to produce any such evidence.

My own experience with thyroid therapy in diabetes suggests that both sides have points in their favor. Evidence at present strongly suggests that the complications of diabetes including atherosclerosis are not due to the diabetes itself but to something independent of diabetes and this may well be thyroid deficiency.

If this is in fact true, then there may be a small danger of aggravating the atherosclerosis by use of a drug such as tolbutamide for the diabetes, for tolbutamide is known to be mildly goitrogenic and suppresses thyroid activity a little, without producing hypothyroidism. But if many diabetics are hypothyroid to begin with and if an oral antidiabetic agent depresses the thyroid a little more, it could aggravate the atherosclerosis.

However, that does not mean that oral antidiabetic drugs should be abandoned. It does mean that we can now stop the complications of diabetes by thyroid therapy and this is essential whether insulin or tolbutamide or any other antidiabetic agent is used. The objection to tolbutamide is overcome with use of thyroid. If atherosclerosis can be controlled with thyroid, an oral antidiabetic tablet is far more attractive to many diabetics than injections of insulin.

Links with the Thyroid

The finding in the University Group Diabetes Program study that 67 percent of deaths in diabetics result from atherosclerosis shows that despite better control of diabetes there has been a rise, not a reduction, in this complication since 1930 when it accounted for slightly under half of diabetic mortality.

The lack of progress indicates that there must be some other reason for arterial degeneration. And since the incidence of deaths from atherosclerosis in the nondiabetic population is almost identical to that in the diabetic, this too suggests that atherosclerosis has nothing to do with diabetes but may have much to do with a factor common to both diabetics and nondiabetics.

Thyroid therapy prevented complications in Dr. Eaton's diabetic patients twenty years ago and has been preventing the same complications in my patients, diabetic and nondiabetic, for twenty-four years.

Not all diabetic patients develop complications. Drs. F. D. W. Ludens and S. N. Franklin of Philadelphia have reported that of 500 diabetic patients followed for twenty years or longer, 11 had no evidence of atherosclerosis.

This small percentage of patients who seem to be immune to arterial damages should be studied carefully to determine how they differ from other diabetics.

I suspect that they have normal thyroid function or perhaps even function that is at the upper limit of normal. By correspondence, I have determined that one diabetic whose disease appeared in childhood and who has been on insulin forty years without evidence of complications has an afternoon temperature that runs a little above normal, suggesting at least normal thyroid function.

All of the diabetic patients I have personally treated to date have run subnormal basal temperatures and have had symptoms of hypothyroidism, and with thyroid therapy they have had not only relief of the hypothyroidism symptoms but have shown no detectable progression in atherosclerosis.

All of the complications of diabetes—including those of the eye (retinopathies), of the nervous system (neuropathies), of the muscles (myopathies), of the joints (arthropathies), of the kidneys (nephropathies), and atherosclerotic gangrene—are seen in hypthyroidism in the absence of diabetes.

In Graz, Austria, a goitrous area for centuries, a large proportion of the population is hypothyroid. I have checked the protocols for 2,400 consecutive autopsies carried out in one year and found that of the total number of amputations required because of gangrene, five of every six were among hypothyroid nondiabetics. It is not diabetes but rather atherosclerosis in both diabetic and nondiabetic that leads to loss of the lower extremities.

Dr. Max Ellenberg of Mount Sinai Hospital in New York City has emphasized for years that most of the complications of diabetes may precede the disturbance in carbohydrate metabolism by many years. He has also been aware of the similarity in symptoms in diabetes and hypothyroidism, but probably because standard thyroid function tests often fail to reveal the hypothyroidism he has not recommended thyroid therapy for diabetics.

I argue emphatically that since so many of the symptoms and complications of hypothyroidism are identical to those of diabetes, every patient with diabetes should have a basal temperature check and, if the temperature is subnormal, a trial of thyroid therapy.

A recent case illustrates the wisdom of this. A sixty-four-year-old man had been diagnosed as diabetic a year before. He had been placed on medication for the diabetes and the diabetes was under good control. Yet he had developed pain, weakness, and atrophy or wasting of the muscles in his left thigh, between knee and hip. He walked with a cane, was uncertain of his balance, had to use strong anti-pain medication day and night. A neurological examination in Phoenix, with nerve conduction and muscle electrical studies, indicated that this was a clear case of diabetic neuropathy.

When his basal temperature was found to be subnormal, he was placed on one grain of thyroid daily. Within a week after starting thyroid, he no longer needed medication for pain; within five weeks, his muscles were strong enough for him to discard his cane, at the end of three months he could walk for miles without difficulty.

There isn't anything miraculous about this. When thyroid function is low, there is, as we have seen earlier, an increase in deposits of mucopolysaccharides that may develop anywhere in connective tissue, including the connective tissue supporting nerves. These abnormal deposits accumulate fluid and may put pressure on a nerve, leading to pain and interference with nerve function. When the nerve supplying a muscle does not function properly, the muscle cannot and, with disuse, the muscle weakens and wastes. With thyroid therapy, the mucopolysaccharide deposits are reduced and the whole process is reversed.

Other symptoms in diabetics—symptoms which are those of hypothyroidism and do not respond to treatment for the diabetes—respond to treatment for the low thyroid function.

The diabetes in a twenty-six-year-old woman who had been on insulin since the age of four was well controlled. But her menstrual periods had never been regular. She had suffered severe menstrual cramps until her pregnancy. The pregnancy ended in miscarriage. She was always tired, had frequent headaches, complained of joint pains. When her basal temperature was found to be subnormal, she was started on a grain of thyroid daily. After three months, she was free of headaches, her periods were regular, she needed less sleep, and her joint pains also had disappeared. There was no change in her insulin requirement.

Diabetes is a hereditary disease. She probably inherited it from her father who was also a diabetic and had died of a heart attack at an early age. Present evidence indicates that his life might have been prolonged with thyroid. The patient's mother is hypothyroid and she may have inherited a proneness to low thyroid function from her mother. Hypothyroidism, too, runs in families.

There may be other reasons why the two conditions so often occur together. In Graz, with its high incidence of hypothyroidism, the incidence of diabetes is twice that found in the United States. Diabetes may be precipitated by infection or other stress. Repeated infection may damage the pancreas. The Austrians have a high rate of infection as do other people with hypothyroidism.

Prediabetes

Since the symptoms of diabetes and those of hypothyroidism are so similar except for the disturbance in carbohydrate metabolism in diabetes, it now seems that we may have, finally, an explanation for the observation of Dr. Ellenberg and others that so-called diabetic complications often precede the diabetes itself.

If the complications are due to hypothyroidism, we can understand why only 20 percent of so-called "prediabetics" ever develop diabetes. Much attenion and effort have gone into diagnosing prediabetes and starting antidiabetic treatment early in hope of stopping atherosclerosis. But the effort has been in vain and it is time for a serious look at the subject of prediabetes.

Prediabetes is a term applied to the state of any individual who has a greater than average probability of developing high blood sugar. This means a probability greater than 2 percent since 2 percent of the American population has overt diabetes.

In 1971, Dr. W. P. U. Jackson of the Department of Medicine of the University of Capetown in South Africa published an extensive review of prediabetes. He listed various categories of people in whom prediabetes might be suspected. If he had been selecting people likely to be suffering from hypothyroidism, he could not have done a better job.

Prediabetes might be suspected, Dr. Jackson noted, in women giving birth to overly large babies. Yet overly large babies were associated with hypothyroidism long before insulin became available and made it possible for many diabetic women to reproduce. A woman whose baby dies at or around the time of birth is suspect for prediabetes. But this has always been and still is associated with thyroid deficiency. In Graz, Austria, with its high rate of hypothyroidism, prenatal deaths in infants accounted for 8.5 percent of total deaths in 1972. And repeated miscarriages, toxemias of pregnancy, and birth of children with congenital anomalies—all listed as possible indicators of prediabetes—are, in fact, classical signs of hypothyroidism.

Obesity is common among diabetics and has been thought of as a predisposing factor. But about 60 percent of thyroid deficient patients are overweight. Since diabetes affects about 2 percent of the population and hypothyroidism may affect 40 percent or more, the odds would favor hypothyroidism as the cause of obesity in diabetes.

Temporary elevation of blood sugar during any stress including pregnancy may be due to hypothyroidism as much as to prediabetes. Repeated attacks of pancreatitis are thought to be one of the causes of diabetes since the infections may destroy the insulin-producing cells of the pancreas. This is true, but susceptibility to infections is frequently due to thyroid deficiency.

Is gout a possible indicator of prediabetes? Gout does occur in diabetics but it is very frequent in hypothyroid patients and thyroid therapy often controls gout without other medications by improving kidney elimination. High blood cholesterol level occurs in diabetics and is supposed to be a possible indicator of the prediabetic state, but high cholesterol is so frequent in hypothyroidism that it has even been used as a diagnostic test for low thyroid function.

The final group of patients likely to become diabetic, according to Jackson's review, are those with atheroscelrosis. But as we have seen, atherosclerosis has been curbed by Dr. Eaton in diabetics by use of thyroid, and I have seen thyroid work the same way in my diabetic patients.

It becomes obvious that all of the criteria of prediabetes reviewed by Jackson fit the picture of hypothyroidism much better. Dr. Jackson has also stated that only 20 percent of prediabetics ever develop overt diabetes. The reason for this, it would seem, is that most of them are hypothyroids rather than candidates for diabetes.

Testing for Diabetes

For many years, the glucose tolerance test has been used to diagnose the diabetic state. It has pitfalls that have been forgotten.

In the first place, a quarter of a pound of sugar on an empty stomach which is taken for the test can hardly be considered normal eating. This is a stress situation in itself. But other stress conditions have been added in the effort to uncover diabetes long before it becomes overt. Many laboratories now add to the sugar some cola which contains caffeine, a compound that releases more sugar from the liver. The liver is supposed to store excess sugar, but now suddenly it gets a shot of caffeine to empty its glucose.

As if this is not abnormal enough, cortisone may be added in an effort to make the glucose tolerance test more sensitive. But cortisone also causes a discharge of glucose from the liver; in fact, continual administration of excess cortisone can be enough in itself to produce diabetes.

Many patients who can handle 100 grams of sugar without evidence of prediabetes are classified as prediabetic or diabetic when they are given two doses of cortisone, one eight and one half hours and the other two hours before the glucose tolerance test. Under these circumstances, the blood sugar will be elevated above the accepted range and it will stay elevated longer.

These are extreme stress conditions and don't necessarily tell us with any great accuracy what the patient can do with a regular diet to which he is accustomed.

Is the huge expenditure for such tests warranted? I seriously doubt it because the tests do not measure pancreatic ability alone but may be obscured by low thyroid function.

Years ago, diabetes was diagnosed when glucose began to spill into the urine. The urgency to detect diabetes at earlier stages, before the spillover occurred, was occasioned by the hope that early treatment for the diabetes could prevent atherosclerosis. But deaths from atherosclerosis in diabetics have continued to climb, paralleling the rise in the nondiabetic population. If atherosclerosis can be combated in both populations by thyroid therapy, more attention ought to be given to early thyroid deficiency diagnosis and less to early detection of diabetes to the exclusion of other factors.

Low thyroid function, we noted above, can obscure the results of tests for diabetes. It can do this with the results not only of the glucose tolerance test but also with those of the simpler and less expensive test in which blood sugar is measured about two hours after a meal. In the normal individual, the blood sugar has returned to near normal level by this time, but in the diabetic it is still elevated. But it may also be elevated with thyroid deficiency.

In hypothyroidism, digestion in the stomach and intestines is delayed. The concentration of acid and enzymes involved in digestion may be diminished. Motility of the gut is reduced and food is propelled more slowly along the tract. Absorption through the intestinal wall is slower.

Obviously, then, the two-hour test for diabetes may not distinguish between diabetes and hypothyroidism because with the delay in digestion in hypothyroidism, blood sugar may still be elevated two hours after a meal.

That glucose tolerance testing also may not distinguish between diabetes and hypothyroidism is illustrated in a study made among Eskimos and reported in *The Canadian Medical Association Journal* in 1968. Glucose tolerance tests were run on 132 Eskimos. They indicated diabetes in over 50 percent of the cases. But diabetes is very rare among Eskimos. This led the investigator to repeat the tests, this time injecting the glucose by vein instead of giving it by mouth. In no case in the second test was there a diabetic response. When the glucose was placed directly in the bloodstream by injection into a vein, the slow absorption in the gut which had suggested diabetes in the first test was bypassed. The slow absorption could have been the result of low thyroid function. And in fact the high incidence of infectious disease and premature death among Eskimos also suggests thyroid deficiency. Basal temperature testing in the Arctic Circle would be very interesting.

Actually, proof that glucose tolerance tests do not distinguish between diabetes and hypothyroidism was furnished fifty years ago by physicians at the St. Thomas Hospital in London. They gave glucose tolerance tests to fifteen patients with myxedema and used only fifty grams of sugar rather than the usual one hundred grams.

In spite of the small quantity of sugar taken, only one of the fifteen patients failed to show elevated blood sugar characteristic of diabetes at the end of two hours. Two of the patients, despite the small amount of sugar used, even spilled some into the urine.

When the patients were treated with thyroid, the glucose tolerance tests showed normal blood sugar levels. Obviously, these patients were not diabetic. The thyroid-deficient patient shows an inability to handle sugar rapidly which is similar to that of the true diabetic and tolerance tests will not differentiate between the two diseases.

"Brittle" Diabetics

Some diabetics are difficult to control. They may swing from insulin reaction one day to sugar in the urine and the appearance of ketone bodies shortly afterward. The ketone bodies are the result of failure to utilize carbohydrates properly which causes the body to draw on its supply of fats to so great an extent that they cannot be handled properly and their incomplete oxidation allows ketones to accumulate in blood and tissues. These are the diabetics who are known as fragile, labile, brittle, volatile, or unstable. It appears that many of them are hypothyroid and that treatment for the hypothyroidism often permits better control of the diabetes.

The somewhat erratic digestion and absorption of food in the hypothyroid patient is one factor. Another is sluggishness of the liver which may occur when thyroid function is low, with the result that stored glucose in the liver is not released properly as blood sugar begins to fall.

There is usually an adequate store of glucose in the liver to last until the next regular meal but, if it is not released, hypoglycemia, or low blood sugar, may develop and call for extra food. Thyroid therapy improves digestion and absorption so that there is a more constant supply of nourishment in the blood; it also sensitizes the liver to the need for glucose release after digestion is complete.

Hypoglycemia

Hypoglycemia occurs in many people who do not test out to be diabetic and who have no family history of diabetes. Some investigators have thought that such people may be prediabetic, but there have been no reports of significant numbers of them later developing overt diabetes.

Hypoglycemia may be tolerated for brief periods without symptoms. But if the blood sugar level remains very low for extended periods, such symptoms as sweating, shakiness, trembling, weakness, anxiety, and, occasionally, seizures or coma may develop.

Treatment usually recommended for hypoglycemia is a diet high in protein and low in carbohydrate, with frequent feedings. I have seen many patients with hypoglycemia who have responded to thyroid therapy. Their symptoms have been ended and they have been able to eat normal diets.

One patient, a forty-four-year-old woman, had gone through what she called a "ten-year nightmare." She had been a secretary and her nightmare had begun when one day, without warning, she passed out at work. She was rushed to a hospital where she recovered from the passing out episode quickly enough. But three days of testing failed to uncover any organic explanation and she was released with the information that she had had a nervous upset and there was nothing to worry about.

But she was emotionally upset, would often cry for no reason, took tranquilizers without relief. Feeling certain that something was wrong, she saw many physicians over the next few years, even a surgeon who referred her to a psychiatrist who insisted that her problem was not mental.

She had two children. She became pregnant again, spilled sugar during her pregnancy, and delivered a stillborn child at term. At that time, a diagnosis of prediabetes was made, but the spilling of sugar stopped almost immediately. Some time later, she was diagnosed as being hypoglycemic. Now carbohydrates were eliminated from her diet which became largely protein. Even small amounts of sugar-containing foods would cause violent headaches. She was given injections of aqueous adrenal extracts, but her condition worsened. She had difficulty in sleeping and experienced periods of severe depression.

When I first saw her, she had had ten years of misery and frustration. Her lifelong history suggested the possibility of hypothyroidism. As a child, she had suffered from repeated respiratory infections with complications, including pneumonia at the age of nine months, and thereafter many severe ear infections.

When her basal temperature proved to be low, she was started on one grain of thyroid daily. Four months later, she began to feel like her old self again. She was able to eat anything she wished, but out of fear tended to avoid sweets. When I insisted that she could eat sweets if she wished to, and gave her a piece of lemon pie to prove it to her, she warned me that she would become upset immediately but she ate the pie, not with enjoyment because of her anxiety but with impunity. And she reported a few weeks later that one day she had indulged a craving that had built up over the years: She ate a pound of chocolates at one sitting.

The Heart of the Problem

More than fifty years after the first insulin injection and despite the development of other antidiabetic drugs, diabetes is still a deadly disease.

But the deadliness lies not in the metabolic abnormality, in the poor utilization of carbohydrates, but rather in the vascular abnormality, in the atherosclerosis which diabetics, like many nondiabetics, develop.

Hypothyroidism, as we have seen, is very much involved in the development of atherosclerosis and the correction of low thyroid function can do much to retard and possibly even prevent the artery disease.

Perhaps we need less emphasis on uncovering pre-diabetes in favor of what could be far more important: emphasis on uncovering low thyroid function at the earliest possible time as a means of combating the atherosclerosis which is the deadly disease and may be at work long before diabetes becomes overt.

And the test for that—a simple basal temperature test—takes little time and involves no expense. It would be wise for everyone to make an occasional basal temperature check—and especially so for everyone with a history of diabetes in the family.

14

The Thyroid, Lung Cancer, and Emphysema

ALTHOUGH THYROID DEFICIENCY, as we have seen, is an important element in the development of heart attacks, hypertension, and the complications of diabetes, its link with cancer is not as clear-cut.

But there are reasons why more attention should be paid to the role of thyroid in the rise in malignancies, particularly lung cancer. That the goiter areas of fifteen countries and four continents consistently show a higher incidence of cancer than adjacent areas of the same countries was pointed out in 1954 by Dr. J. G. C. Spencer, a pathologist at the Frenahay Hospital in Bristol, England. And hypothyroidism is far more common in the goiter areas than in the adjacent regions.

Austria, a country with a high incidence of goiter, has the highest incidence of cancer of any country reporting malignancies.

241

It is also a fact that if one tries to transplant a cancer from one rat to another, the grafted malignancy will seldom "take" unless the thyroid gland is removed beforehand.

The Rise in Lung Cancer

Although malignant tumors have been known all throughout history, they were relatively infrequent 150 years ago. Because better health records were kept in England in the last century than in the rapidly expanding United States, and because the population was more stable in Britain, the increase in cancer can be traced better there.

It was just before the turn of the century that British physicians began to feel deeply concerned about cancer. In 1898, one of them, Dr. Roger Williams, in a report in the journal *Lancet*, noted that unless something could be done to stop the rise in cancer, it would soon be as lethal as typhoid, smallpox, and tuberculosis combined, and these were the leading causes of death at the time.

He traced the increase in cancer mortality from 1840 to 1890 and found that in the fifty-year period, the rate had gone from 17 deaths per 100,000 population to 88, an increase of more than five fold. Today, the rate is more than 150 deaths per 100,000.

In 1898, Dr. Williams blamed environmental factors, as we still largely do today. He advocated, as preventive measures, more fresh air, more exercise, and more vegetables in the diet since meat consumption had doubled during the fifty-year period. Undoubtedly, had cigarette smoking been fashionable at the time, Dr. Williams would have included it as a culprit not only in lung cancer but in all cancer.

Lung cancer today is one of the leading causes of death. According to the American Cancer Sociery, 79,000 new cases now occur each year. The malignancy today is fifteen times more frequent than forty years ago. The highest incidence occurs between the ages of fifty and sixty years. Less than 1 percent of lung cancers develop in people under thirty; approximately 10 percent occur in people after age seventy.

The increase in lung cancer has been blamed on air pollution and cigarette smoking. Yet a clue which has had little attention lies in the fact that just as the incidence of heart attacks has risen as deaths from infectious diseases have declined, so has the incidence of lung cancer.

I have noted earlier in this book the valuable records to be found in Graz, Austria. In 1960, Dr. Max Ratzenhofer of the Pathological Institute of the University of Graz and I analyzed data taken from 26,546 autopsies done in Graz from 1944 through 1958 and reported the results in *The Journal of the American Medical Association*.

We found the same increase in lung cancer as reported from other areas. In 1944, 22 cases of lung cancer were found in 1,820 postmortem examinations. In 1958, there were 83 cases in 2,249 autopsies.

During this interval of fifteen years, mortality from tuberculosis also showed remarkable changes. In 1944, the 1,820 autopsies included 236 deaths from tuberculosis. By 1955, out of 1,965 autopsies, tuberculosis was the reason for death in only 58 cases and in this same year, for the first time, more deaths were recorded from cancer of the lung than from tuberculosis. The same was true for succeding years.

Other important changes took place during the fifteen-year period. For one thing, the average age of persons who died from tuberculosis increased. In 1944, the average age at death had been thirty-eight years; by 1957, it was fifty-four years. In other words, the tubercular patient was living longer and approaching the "cancer age" before death.

A second change was the frequent association of tuberculosis with cancer. For years, it had been generally believed that malignancies are not common in patients with tuberculosis. In Graz, in 1946, for the first time, tuberculosis was found in bronchial cancer. Seven of fifty-two patients dying of lung cancer also had tuberculosis. The peak was reached in 1948, when 21 percent of the patients with lung cancer had associated tuberculosis. There have been fewer cases of the two diseases in the same patient since because, apparently, as the incidence of tuberculosis decreases, there is less likelihood of the association.

A review of the medical literature shows that lung cancer began to increase in incidence in Europe about the time the incidence of tuberculosis began to fall. In Manchester, England, the phenomenon was first noted in 1871; in Dresden, Germany, in 1891. By 1895, when the German physician, Kurt Wolf, realized that an epidemic of lung cancer was beginning, he found that 42 percent of his lung cancer patients had active tuberculosis. This was at a time when sanitarium care was prolonging the life of tubercular patients. Wolf felt that the tuberculosis was causing the lung cancer. A more rational explanation today is that the same patient is susceptible to either disease.

Many investigators have reported an association between tuberculosis and lung cancer. Only one study will be mentioned. At the VA Hospital in Memphis, Tennessee, among 11,000 patients with tuberculosis, 650 also developed lung cancer. In the VA study, patients with tuberculosis proved to be twenty times more susceptible to lung cancer than the general population.

Is the Thyroid Involved?

The data from Graz and elsewhere suggest that one factor in the increase in lung cancer is that persons who previously would have died from infectious disease are alive today.

As we have seen, low thyroid function plays a significant role in increasing susceptibility to infectious disease, and it may very well play a similar role in increasing susceptibility to lung cancer.

It could be only coincidence that among thousands of patients I have placed on thyroid therapy, not one has developed lung cancer and there have been only six deaths due to malignancies of any kind while in a similar number of people in the general population about twenty deaths from cancer would have been expected.

An explanation for the role of thyroid deficiency in cancer may lie in the growing evidence that viruses are linked to some cancers. It is firmly established that hypothyroid patients—and hypothyroid animals—are unusually susceptible to infections and that thyroid therapy increases their resistance to infectious agents, including the viruses responsible for the common cold and influenza.

The occurrence of these and other infections is markedly curtailed, and even the elderly do not need immunization against influenza if their thyroid function, as determined by basal temperature, is brought up to the normal range.

It would seem worthwhile, as a possible prophylaxis against cancer, particularly lung cancer, to check the basal temperature of all people, especially those with susceptibility to infections, and to correct low thyroid function when it is found.

There is no question that they would enjoy better health day in and day out. And it could well be that a study following such patients over many years would show a marked reduction in incidence of lung cancer.

Emphysema

Emphysema, a chronic progressive disease of the lungs, is another disease which, like lung cancer, has become increasingly common in recent years. It now causes a significant number of deaths each year. In the United States, reported deaths from emphysema rose from 2,300 in 1945 to 15,000 in 1962 and are still on the increase. In Graz, Austria, a rise of 372 percent occurred between 1930 and 1970.

Emphysema, moreover, ranks as the major single

cause of disability of pulmonary origin, producing shortness of breath and wheezing that progressively limit activity and too often advance to the point of virtually complete invalidism.

Because, as we shall see, repeated infections constitute a major factor in the development of the disease, any method for increasing resistance to infectious disease might be expected to reduce the incidence of emphysema. And since thyroid deficiency is accompanied by lowered resistance while correction of the deficiency raises resistance, this would seem to be an approach worth consideration.

And among thyroid-treated patients in my experience, emphysema has been conspicuous by its absence. Not one such patient has developed serious emphysema.

The Disease

There has been some confusion about emphysema and chronic bronchitis. Actually, both problems usually coexist and are often described together under such names as "chronic obstructive lung disease" (COLD) and "chronic obstructive pulmonary emphysema" (COPE).

The word "obstructive" refers to the changes that take place in the bronchi and bronchioles, the passages carrying air to the lungs where oxygen is exchanged for carbon dioxide. The bronchi and bronchioles have cells that produce mucus to trap foreign material. Normally the mucus is washed up almost continuously to the throat where it is swallowed or eliminated through the mouth and nose.

When proper elimination of mucus is hampered, the

retained mucus narrows the air passages. As a result, greater force is needed to expel air. This puts abnormal strain on the alveoli, the thin-walled chambers of the lungs where oxygen and carbon dioxide are exchanged. They become overdistended because of the abnormally high pressure in the lungs which the patient must produce in order to force air through the narrowed airways, in effect having to squeeze air from his chest.

The stage when mucus accumulates in the airways and the accumulation is accompanied by narrowing and inflammation of the airways is called chronic bronchitis. The stage when the alveoli are compromised is called emphysema.

During the chronic bronchitis stage, there may be persistent cough and sputum production. It is when the alveoli become compromised that shortness of breath develops.

In some cases, chronic bronchitis does not go on to produce emphysema, but these are the exceptions rather that the rule. Similarly, some people may suffer predominantly from emphysema with little or none of the changes of chronic bronchitis but, again, they are the exceptions.

It may take as few as five years or as many as thirty years for shortness of breath and wheezing to develop. Cough is hard and tiring and may be triggered by any exertion, even talking.

The chest is overinflated and in some cases may remain fixed so that there is no rise and fall with breathing in and out. Accessory muscles have to be used for breathing and they undergo great strain, the head moving with each inhalation.

Cigarette smoking, air pollution, and exposure to industrial fumes have been blamed for either causing or exacerbating emphysema. That they can exacerbate the problem is clear enough; whether they play a significant role in causing it is still not definitely known.

It is also clearly established that respiratory infection exacerbates emphysema. And it is agreed that the course of emphysema is determined largely by the frequency with which acute episodes of bronchial infection occur.

The Role of Infections

But infections play a major role in causing chronic bronchitis and emphysema in the first place. Almost invariably, emphysema patients I have seen have had histories of repeated infections. Almost any kind of infection, it appears, may play a role. One that may well deserve special note here is chronic sinusitis, called "catarrh" by our forefathers. And it may persist unnoticed for years.

Nasal stuffiness or postnasal drip may come to be accepted by the patient as a way of life after no physician seems to be able to do anything about it. Not infrequently, ear, nose, and throat specialists may deny that sinusitis is present since there are no shadows on X-rays, yet the patient is constantly clearing his throat as mucus and pus drain down over the pharynx. The throat, not in the region of the tonsils but lower down, may become sore, and the irritation may lead to cough. Especially after a cold, many people complain of a cough that persists for months.

Often, the lymph glands on either side of the neck may

become inflamed and sore as the result of toxic sub-
stances draining down from infected sinuses through the
lymph channels. Sometimes the drainage may even set
up a neuritis in the upper chest which may be confused
with pleurisy or even angina, the chest pain that often
accompanies heart disease.

It is often possible to relieve the neuritis in a few days
with either an injection of vitamin B-12 or by taking
brewer's yeast tablets, which are full of B vitamins, by
mouth.

And it is often possible, too, to overcome a sinus or
other infection with antibiotics. But the antibiotics do
nothing to prevent recurrences and each infection damages the lungs a little more and the effects are cumula-
tive. If the patient survives long enough, a full-blown case
of emphysema results.

Emphysema has been found even in babies suffering
from severe infection. The thin-walled alveoli in the
lungs are very delicate and have to be for carbon dioxide
and oxygen to be transferred through them. They are
easily damaged. At autopsy, babies dying of infection
may be found to have ruptured alveoli and air escaped
into the interstitial tissues. This is called interstitial emphysema.

Thus in the autopsy protocols at Graz for the year
1930, case #7 was a five-month-old baby who died of
meningitis and who had interstitial emphysema. The
toxins from the infection had injured the alveoli, causing
emphysema, but the fatal meningitis prevented further
development of the emphysema.

Protocol #94 for the same year was for a year-old girl

who died of dysentery; again interstitial emphysema was present. Protocol #461 was for a baby boy who died at six days with pneumonia. Interstitial emphysema was present.

Without the autopsies, it would never have been known that emphysematous changes can begin so early. If these children had recovered from their infections, the tiny holes in the alveoli would have healed, the scar tissue formed for the healing would have been incapable of normal transfer of gases, and the way would have been paved for the development of adult emphysema.

It is the reduction in deaths from infection in childhood and adulthood that is the major factor in the rise of emphysema. Where in years gone by those susceptible to infections died early, antibiotics available since 1945 have saved millions who would otherwise have succumbed, and for the first time in history emphysema has become a common disease.

I spent one summer vacation in Graz studying the history of emphysema there as indicated by the autopsies. Every case for the years studied in which there was any mention of emphysema was checked.

Since emphysema is generally considered to be a degenerative disease, it might be expected that patients dying of degenerative diseases would show more emphysema than others.

But this was not the case. Among patients dying of infectious diseases, 90 percent had some degree of emphysema. Among those dying of cancer, 35 percent had some degree of emphysema. And emphysema was present in 28 percent of those dying of other degenerative diseases and in 21 percent of those killed in accidents.

One of the most dramatic examples of the role of infections in emphysema is provided by the autopsy record at Graz of a twenty-one-year-old man whose emphysema was as severely advanced as that of a seventy-year-old. From the age of six, he had been hospitalized repeatedly with severe infections. He had had recurrent attacks of bronchitis. Chronic tonsillitis had led to myocarditis—inflammation of the heart muscle. He had had three attacks of pneumonia and his final hospital admission was for a fourth episode of pneumonia. Two weeks before his death, he developed great difficulty in breathing, cyanosis or blueness, and swelling of the legs. The autopsy showed hemorrhagic bronchitis, pleural adhesions, and far advanced emphysema; so advanced, in fact, that it had led to heart enlargement and congestive heart failure. In fifteen years of repeated infections, emphysema had progressed to the point of no return, a process that usually requires fifty years.

The best approach to emphysema is prevention. That means eliminating infections in the young and maintaining high resistance to them throughout life.

Still, considerable help can be found even after early symptoms appear. As soon as shortness of breath is noticed, a thorough check should be made for the presence of any infection, however low-grade or subtle it may be. The infection should be treated. If thyroid function is low, as indicated by basal temperature, thyroid therapy should be used to correct the low function and to bolster resistance to infection.

A sixty-three-year-old man came in for a routine examination. He had no major complaints. He had retired from business but had bought a small farm and was actively working it. His history indicated some tendency to infections earlier in life, an attack of pneumonia at age thirty-eight, a strep throat infection four years later.

At examination, it was apparent that he had nasal congestion and postnasal drip indicative of chronic sinusitis. His basal temperature was low and thyroid therapy was started to correct his mild hypothyroidism and help his resistance. At the time, there were no indications of emphysema and no therapy was advised for his low-grade sinusitis except thryoid.

A few months later, however, he discovered while doing a bit of mountain climbing that he became markedly short of breath. We then instituted active treatment with nasal decongestants for the sinusitis because the chronic sinus drainage was aggravating a developing emphysema still in early stages. Over the past five years, while there has been no improvement in the emphysema, there has been no deterioration. Present indications are that the emphysema is static and he has a normal life expectancy and can continue to farm as he wishes and enjoy an active life.

Twenty-two years ago, a salesman, then aged forty-five, developed shortness of breath because of emphysema. As a child he had been susceptible to infections, including repeated ear abscesses. On examination, he was found to have chronic sinusitis which was treated. His blood chemistry showed a cholesterol of 381, suggesting subnormal thyroid function. A basal temperature check confirmed the hypothyroidism and he was placed on thyroid treatment. His cholesterol level came down and has remained at normal value. Now, at sixty-seven, he leads an active life, gets short of breath only with overexertion. There is no evidence of any progress of the emphysema.

A woman now in her seventies had been susceptible to respiratory infections all of her life. She had suffered from severe menstrual cramps until the birth of her first child. After the arrival of her second child, she had spent thirteen months in a tuberculosis sanitarium. While there, her sinusitis bothered her more than the tuberculosis, although it was necessary to have one lung collapsed.

When she was thirty-seven, it became apparent that some of her problems were due to hypothyroidism and thyroid therapy was started. Her lung healed more rapidly thereafter. Thyroid therapy has been continued ever since and she has had much better resistance to infections.

Shortness of breath upon more than moderate exertion became apparent at about the age of sixty-five, but she still carries on household duties and in addition works several hours each day outside the home. Her performance, in fact, is far better than that of the average person of her age in spite of her latent emphysema.

It seems certain that without thyroid therapy to reduce her susceptibility to infections, including very severe ones, this woman would have been a candidate for early crippling emphysema. It was fortunate that her thyroid therapy was started long before it was realized that emphysema is one of the complications of chronic infection.

No one will deny that environmental factors such as polluted air and smoking will aggravate emphysema, once it is well established. But inheritance seems to be more important than environment, especially inheritance of low thyroid function and with it a proclivity for infectious disease.

Among many hundreds of patients treated with thyroid and observed for many years in the study to determine whether thyroid therapy can help to prevent heart attacks, not a single case of emphysema has developed even though there has been no restriction of smoking. It would appear that thyroid therapy can be effective prophylaxis for emphysema.

15

The Thyroid and Obesity: The Real—and Surprising—Connections

THE THYROID HAS MUCH TO DO with obesity—but not in the way many people have long thought. Loading in thyroid when thyroid function is normal is hardly the answer to obesity. The results of such treatment can be even worse than the effects of obesity. If thyroid function is low, correcting it with thyroid therapy will help—but again this is not the whole answer.

What is needed for overcoming obesity is proper diet —not what is generally considered to be proper diet but effective diet for losing weight—and good thyroid function.

The chances are that what you read in this chapter is going to surprise you, to upset many notions you have long heard bruited about, and if it does surprise you and you have a weight problem, the surprise will be a gratifying one and it is far from inconceivable that for the first time in your life you will be able to reduce effectively and painlessly and maintain your desired weight effectively and painlessly.

The Human Guinea Pigs

My interest in obesity was sharpened soon after I finished medical school when I became an assistant professor of Medicine at the University of Illinois, working under the late Dr. Robert W. Keeton.

Dr. Keeton had been interested in obesity for many years. When I arrived, he was particularly anxious to see just how important the mysterious glands of internal secretion—the endocrines—were in obesity.

At that time, it was common practice for physicians to inject extracts of the pituitary gland for weight reduction. It was known that some of the preparations from the pituitary would mobilize stored material in the body and produce elevated blood sugar levels. The theory behind the injections was that they would help control appetite. Since I had a background of several years of work in the endocrine field, Dr. Keeton assigned the project to me.

A three-bed ward was available where volunteer obese patients could stay as long as necessary for the investigation. This was in 1938, near the end of the depression, and help was furnished by the federal government under the Works Progress Administration program. We had a dietitian available to cater to the whims of the volunteers, preparing for them anything they wanted to eat, weighing out their selections for each meal, calculating the proportions of carbohydrate, protein, and fat, and weighing again anything they left uneaten on their trays.

For a period of three months, she kept a precise record of everything they put into their mouths. The purpose was to find out if possible from their eating habits and whims how they got into their present shape. And their shapes were something to write home about. A total of thirteen patients were studied. The champion was a middle-aged woman with a height of exactly 60 inches and an abdominal measurement of 72 inches. She was literally "Mrs. 5 x 6" and weighed 350 pounds. There were two rolls of fat around her abdomen, one just above the pelvis and the other around the stomach area. The two rolls touched each other and resembled two tractor tires around a barrel.

With one exception, all of the volunteers weighed over 300 pounds. The runt of the bunch weighed only 295, but she was included because she was only eighteen years old and was brought into the outpatient department because she could no longer get under a bed. She had been fat all of her life and was very embarrassed about it—to the point where as soon as company would come to visit at the farm in southern Illinois, she would scoot under the bed and stay there until they left. The problem was to put higher legs under the bed or else reduce her. She was kept longer than any of the others but her problem was solved. She served as a guinea pig for thirteen months.

What They Ate

One factor common to all of our volunteer guinea pigs was the selection of a diet high in carbohydrates. They kept their protein intake moderate; they avoided fat like the plague. There might be three hard rolls on a tray but never a smidgen of butter. Butter, in their philosophy, was fattening. All fat, as they saw it, was the larding factor. They trimmed it off their meat and they avoided other foods high in fat which they couldn't remove. It became obvious that a high carbohydrate diet had to be considered a causative factor in their obesity.

For those of you who grew up on a farm, this information should be no news. For centuries, farmers have reduced protein intake, eliminated most of the fat, and shoveled in cereals to fatten animals for market. Unfortunately, physicians seldom go to the farm for medical information or we might long ago have had the answer to obesity. The tall corn of Iowa and pork production go hand in hand. The eating habits and metabolism of human and hog are so similar that they could well be embarrassing to the hog.

We shall talk about alterations in diet presently, but it will be well to clear up, first, the role of pituitary injections in weight loss.

After a satisfactory reducing diet had been worked out and the volunteers had been placed on it, pituitary injections were alternated with placebo or inert injections. From the weight loss which was relatively steady, it was impossible to tell when the pituitary injections were stopped and the placebo injections were begun.

There can be little doubt that injections given in a private office may be helpful. If a patient is on a diet and must call at the office several times a week for a shot with a dull needle, he or she is likely to be more conscientious about the diet and weight loss is likely. But under the circumstances of our study, with the only diet available to the patient being one that was carefully weighed out, the pituitary injections had no beneficial effect.

Fats and Carbohydrates

In most biological systems, if a certain combination of circumstances produces a reaction, reversing the circumstances will often reverse the reaction. This has proven to be true in the case of weight management.

Trial and error probably led the farmer to eliminate fat from the diet of animals he wanted to fatten. No one will deny that it works.

And there are sound physiological facts to explain why it does. Fat empties out of the stomach slowly. This has been demonstrated repeatedly by mixing various types of foods with barium. The barium allows one to check on stomach contents periodically by X-ray or fluoroscope. It takes much longer for a fat meal to empty out of the stomach than it does for a carbohydrate meal containing the same amount of calories.

When a hog fills its stomach with corn, it promptly takes a nap. But in approximately ninety minutes, it is awakened by hunger contractions signaling that it is time to eat again. The hog hurries back to the trough for more food, and it is quite true that a little pig eats so much that it makes a hog of itself. What is important in weight control is the time that food spends in the stomach and intestinal tract. Carbohydrates are easier to digest, are readily absorbed and stored in the liver or in muscles, thereby making room as well as creating a quick demand for more.

One of Dr. Keeton's contributions to the understanding of obesity was the demonstration that all types of foodstuffs, when consumed in amounts providing the same number of calories, contribute equally to weight gain or loss. Working with swine, for example, he kept protein intake constant and, using a diet 20 percent below what was needed for weight maintenance, showed that weight loss was exactly the same whether the remainder of the calories was provided by fat or carbohydrate. As long as the caloric intake was the same, the loss was just as fast when fat was used as it was when carbohydrates were used.

But what the swine could not tell us was how they felt. The fat meals would empty out of their stomachs more slowly and they may have been more comfortable, with fewer hunger pangs.

While my volunteers were demonstrating their propensity for choosing high-carbohydrate foods, one of my fraternity brothers was studying high-fat diets in rats. He was working for one of the packing companies in Chicago that was looking for a use for the excess fat from slaughtered animals. He found that old fat rats lost the excess of fat in their abdomens on a diet with a higher than normal fat content. He suggested that I try such a diet on my pachyderm volunteers. I decided to follow his suggestion but I wasn't really prepared for what happened.

The WPA dietitian prepared a diet containing 50 grams of carbohydrate, 70 grams of protein, and 90 grams of fat, adding up to about 1,300 calories a day. For breakfast, this meant two eggs with bacon, ham, or sausage; two ounces of fruit juice; beverage with cream if desired; but no sugar or toast. Luncheon and dinner consisted of a portion of fat meat, a vegetable with butter or oleo on it, a salad with generous salad dressing, a glass of milk, and a small serving of fresh fruit for dessert.

The vegetable and fruits were chosen from those

Table 2

Reducing Diet

DO EAT FATS: *REDUCE* SWEETS AND STARCHES

BREAKFAST

2 eggs
3 strips bacon, sausage, or ham
2 oz. fruit juice—unsweetened
coffee or tea, cream (optional) without sugar

LUNCH AND DINNER (EACH)
One serving meat, fish or fowl
Vegetable with pat of butter or oleo
Salad with abundance of dressing
One serving fresh fruit
One glass of milk, tea, or coffee

If weight is not lost, reduce the quantity eaten.

AVOID: Bread, crackers, pancakes, waffles, potatoes, rice macaroni, spaghetti, corn, bananas, pie, cake, cookies, ice cream, sherbets, candy, colas, raisins, Jell-o, and all starches, sugars, and cereals.

ADD: 3 brewer's yeast tablets daily.

lower in carbohydrate or on occasion a smaller quantity of those with higher carbohydrate content was used. Without any bread or cereals, the vitamin B content of the diet was low and the diet was supplemented with three or more brewer's yeast tablets daily.

The accompanying tables show the reducing diet used with the volunteers and since then for many hundreds of patients, along with a list of common vegetables and their carbohydrate content.

Table 3

Percentages of Carbohydrates in Vegetables and Fruits

EAT SPARINGLY OF 15 PERCENT AND 20 PERCENT GROUPS

5 PERCENT VEGETABLES

Asparagus	Kohlrabi
Bean sprouts	Lettuce
Broccoli	Okra
Cabbage	Olives (ripe)
Cauliflower	Peppers
Celery	Pumpkin
Chard	Radishes
Chinese cabbage	Spinach
Cucumber	String beans
Eggplant	Summer squash
Endive	Tomatoes
Greens (beets)	Turnips
Greens (mustard)	Watercress

10 PERCENT VEGETABLES
Beets
Brussel sprouts
Carrots
Dandelion greens
Leeks
Olives (green)
Onions
Rutabagas
Winter squash

15 PERCENT VEGETABLES
Artichokes
Oyster plant
Parsnips
Peas

20 PERCENT VEGETABLES
Beans (kidney, lima, navy)
Corn
Potatoes
Hominy

5 PERCENT FRUIT
Avocado
Honeydew melon
Muskmelon
Strawberries
Watermelon

10 PERCENT FRUIT
Blackberries
Grapefruit
Oranges
Peaches
Tangerines

15 PERCENT FRUIT
Apples
Apricots
Blueberries
Cherries (tart)
Grapes
Huckleberries
Loganberries
Mulberries
Pears
Pineapple
Plums
Raspberries

20 PERCENT FRUIT
Bananas
Cherries (sweet)
Figs (fresh)
Grape juice
Prunes (fresh)

OTHER ITEMS HIGH IN FAT
(Eat sparingly for snacks)
Cheese
Olives
Avocado
Nuts
Peanut butter

The volunteers were hospitalized for weeks. They lost weight steadily, averaging a 10-pound loss per month But the astonishing thing was acceptance of the menu. Every one of the volunteers was comfortable and had no need to fight hunger pangs. In fact, it was not unusual for them to leave some of their 1,300 calories.

The eighteen-year-old girl who weighed 295 pounds to begin with, remained on this diet in the hospital for nine additional months. Her total weight loss was 110 pounds. She lost most of it from between her knees and shoulders. Her abdomen and hips showed the most remarkable loss. And her face was not drawn and haggard as is the case so often with people losing so much weight.

Eleven months after she went back home, she was kind enough to send me a snapshot. She now weighed 137 pounds, was well proportioned, and her face still was not drawn. She had lost 48 more pounds at home on her own, knowing what to eat. She no longer needed a bed under which to hide from company. The course of her life had been changed.

I have prescribed this diet for patients for more than thirty-five years and the results have been consistent. There have been no patients who did not lose weight as long as they stayed on the diet. It is a convenient diet since it contains food that might be prepared for the rest of the family.

When the desired amount of weight has been lost, enough carbohydrate can be added to the diet to maintain weight at that level and that usually means adding a piece of toast for breakfast and a dessert at the other two meals. There is none of the sudden great shift in eating with starvation or crash diets, and it is necessary only to drop the carbohydrates again if weight begins to accumulate.

Added Evidence

Actually as early as 1929, two Pittsburgh investigators, Drs. F. A. Evans and J. M. Strang, had reported a study in which they used a high-fat diet for weight reduction. They worked with 111 patients and their diet was low enough in carbohydrates to produce ketosis. It consisted of 29 grams of fat, 60 grams of protein, and 45 grams of carbohydrate and contained only 681 calories. Most of the patients lost four pounds a week for the first four weeks, then more than three pounds a week for the next four weeks. The patients were enthusiastic about the results. After the fourth day, only one complained of hunger.

That loss of weight was faster than that on the 1,300-calorie diet suggested above, but with the latter, ketosis is avoided by the extra carbohydrate and the change in eating pattern is not so rigorous.

In 1944, Dr. A. B. Anderson of the University of Glasgow reported satisfactory weight loss with a 600- to 900-calorie high-fat diet containing enough carbohydrate to prevent ketosis.

In 1952, two reports, one from Michigan State University and the other from Cornell, told of results with diets in which over half of the calories came from fat. In the Michigan State study, 1,500 calories daily were allowed and the losses in sixteen weeks ranged from 17 to 34 pounds. At Cornell, fewer calories were used and the average weight loss was 17 pounds in eight and one half weeks. In both studies, appetites were satisfied and there was no ketosis since enough carbohydrate was in the diet.

About the same time, Dr. Alfred W. Pennington at the Du Pont Company was recommending a reducing diet high in fat. In an English study reported in *Lancet* in 1956, investigators reported that weight was lost much faster on a high-fat diet than on a high-protein diet even though the calorie content was the same.

It appears from many studies that weight loss is more rapid and patients better satisfied with a high-fat diet. Although it has long been thought by some that fat in the diet should be reduced since the calorie content per gram of fat is about twice that of carbohydrate or protein, this is offset by the longer time fat spends in the stomach and the reduction in appetite.

There seems little doubt that a high-fat diet reduces the appetite through the slower release from the stomach of a fatty meal and by avoiding the excessive rise in blood sugar so common with high carbohydrate intake. A high sugar level in the blood causes a release of insulin into the bloodstream which must be countered by more glucose.

That insulin itself can be a potent factor in increasing appetite was demonstrated in rats at the time I was at the University of Illinois in 1938. When long-acting insulin was injected in the animals at twelve-hour intervals, the rats reached weights two to three times those for normal adult rats. Undoubtedly, the accumulation of fat was due to persistent low blood sugar. If food were removed from the cage for one hour, some of the animals would die in hypoglycemic convulsions.

Proof that a diet high in fat will depress appetite was obtained several years ago in studies with hogs. No animal has a greater appetite than the hog whose ability to convert feed to edible meat exceeds that of all other animals. The hog's diet ordinarily is very low in fat and high in carbohydrate. Since fat had been shown to depress the appetite in humans, I thought it would be worthwhile seeing what it would do in hogs.

Hogs are very fond of fat and can smell it if it is concealed in a pocket. Walking through a feedlot with a chunk of suet in one's pocket attracts a squealing bunch of followers much in the manner of the Pied Piper of Hamlin.

When the amount of either beef tallow or lard was gradually increased until some of the fat was available to the hogs at all times, the quantity of food eaten was reduced to the point that the animals stopped gaining weight. A diet that will depress a hog's appetite will control almost anyone's craving for food.

But Is It Safe?

If a diet high in fat is valuable for weight control, what of its safety? For the past twenty-five years, the alleged danger of fats and especially saturated fats has been highly publicized. The time has come to correct the erroneous allegation.

The evidence that atherosclerosis might be related to diet was circumstantial, as we have seen in Chapter 12. In the absence of any other apparent approach to the artery disease problem, diet manipulation became popular.

Yet, as we have seen upon critical examination the evidence incriminating diet does not stand up. It was not, for example, the fluctuations in diet during World War II that accounted for the reduction in heart attacks at that time but rather the upsurge of deaths from infectious diseases which reduced opportunities for heart attacks to strike.

And as we have seen, too, the level of cholesterol in the blood is related to the level of thyroid function and the correction of low thyroid function reduces elevated cholesterol level to normal range.

If diet has any role in atherosclerosis and heart attacks, it is minor compared to other factors. Yet diet manipulation has been a major factor in the rise of obesity. With fat in the diet restricted, many of the calories that formerly came from fat were replaced by calories from carbohydrates. But carbohydrates empty out of the stomach rapidly and increase appetite. In countries where food is scarce and much more energy expenditure is needed to obtain what is available, stomachs have been conditioned to not being full all the time and obesity is no problem. But in advanced societies where delicacies are abundant and refrigerators keep leftovers edible, the hog's eating habits are mimicked and weight accumulates. And all the more so because snacks are high in carbohydrates and the stomach is soon empty of them and calling for more.

Now that it is clear that dietary fat is not responsible for the rise in heart attacks in the twentieth century, it is possible to include more fat in the diet to help control obesity effectively and safely.

Mother Nature designed milk to promote the growth and development of the newborn. More that 50 percent of the calories in milk come from fat. It seems unreasonable that fat should be dangerous to health, or life would have been snuffed out long ago.

But we are concerned here with obesity already present and how to get rid of it, and it appears that a high-fat diet may be the most effective method of weight reduction. It even offers results comparable to those obtained with a no-calorie diet—and without the expense and inconvenience of the latter.

Starvation and Nonstarvation

Total starvation has been recommended for weight reduction for people for whom obesity is a major handicap and who are unable to reduce by other means. Because weakness and low blood pressure commonly occur with total starvation, hospitalization is required.

One of the pioneers in using total starvation for combating obesity, Dr. Thomas G. Duncan of the University of Pennsylvania, has reported that some 1,300 persons from all walks of life have been treated with a no-calorie diet. In the regimen, patients receive only coffee, tea, water, or another no-calorie beverage. Within twenty-four hours, the carbohydrate stores of the body are exhausted and ketone bodies appear in the urine in large quantities. This is due to the mobilization of stored body fat for energy and the amount of ketone bodies liberated during the mobilization is so large that they cannot be metabolized and escape into the urine. Usually, weight loss over a two-week period is 18 pounds, with some of it due to loss of water.

A major trouble with the total starvation approach is that it calls for more hospital beds and more doctors to supervise the regimen than are available to fill the need if total starvation is the only effective answer to obesity.

Suppose, however, that a ketogenic diet used at home is able to achieve the same end. Some years ago I developed, and subsequently published, a report in 1965 on, such a diet. Ketosis could be obtained simply by eliminating most of the carbohydrates while allowing sufficient amounts of protein and fats to provide energy to carry on normal activities and to permit normal body-maintenance processes to continue.

Breakfast included bacon and eggs and a peeled orange to furnish a vitamin necessary for health of blood vessels. During the rest of the day, only a liquid eggnog was consumed and it could be consumed as desired. It was made by adding one egg to each pint of whipping cream (20 percent fat), with vanilla, nutmeg, and non-caloric sweetener added to suit individual taste, and the mixture blended in an electric mixer or shaken in a fruit jar. Usually a quart of the formula would be more than enough for a day; most people consumed no more than two-thirds of it. It could be carried to work in a thermos bottle.

This may not seem very appetizing, but it is cheaper and more practical than hospitalization. Ketone bodies appear in the urine within 24 hours and appetite is markedly depressed. A feeling of well-being develops in most cases in a few days and the diet could be continued for weeks if the monotony could be tolerated. However, some people cannot tolerate a sudden change to so much fat and diarrhea may develop.

The diet was recommended only to avoid hospitalization and total starvation in the most difficult cases of
obesity. It is much more appropriate to use the 1,300-
calorie diet outlined earlier and containing enough carbohydrates to avoid ketosis.

Is the appearance of ketone bodies in the urine a
hazard? So some have believed and yet they have forgotten the work of the explorers, Vilhjalmur Stefansson and
Karsten Andersen, in 1929 and 1930. When they returned from the Artic and told of Eskimos eating nothing
but fat caribou meat all winter, running ketone bodies in
the urine all the time without apparent harm, and able to
work rigorously and expend great amounts of energy,
many physicians refused to believe the story.

Both explorers then volunteered to be hospitalized in
New York City for a year while they ate nothing but fat
meat and complete studies were made on them. Their
diet was composed of 2,522 celories a day, of which more
than 75 percent were supplied by fat.

Both men lost about 6 pounds as the result of less water
retention. No abnormalities appeared in their blood
chemistry; their blood pressures remained unchanged;
although they took no supplementary vitamins, no vitamin deficiencies appeared. Both continually excreted
large quantities of ketone bodies yet both appeared in
excellent health at the end of the year. The study indicated that at least over a period of a year a ketogenic diet
produces no undesirable effects.

In defense of high fat diets, the experience of a New
York City cardiologist some years ago is worth noting. He
had many patients with heart disease who needed to
reduce and he had only one diet which consisted of

one-half pound of fat meat three times a day. Not only did his patients lose weight successfully but they suffered no deleterious effects and their heart function improved. Personal experience has confirmed that it is possible to lose weight on this quantity of meat and, of course, with no carbohydrate in the diet, ketosis will occur. If this is not harmful to people with failing hearts, one would not expect any trouble in people with normal hearts.

High Protein and Thyroid Function

For many years, the standard diet prescribed by many physicians has been one with high protein content and little fat. The basis for it has been the fact that there are more calories per unit of weight in fat than in other foodstuffs.

What was not realized was the effect of a diet high in protein on thyroid function—which explains why many patients have failed to lose weight on as few as 800 calories a day of such a diet and have been accused of cheating on their diet when, in fact, they did no cheating.

In experiments conducted on myself, I found that when the intake of carbohydrate and fat was kept low and I ate mostly veal and turkey, diarrhea soon developed and I had feelings of malaise and illness.

On the other hand, when the diet was changed so that it was low in fat but high in protein and with enough carbohydrate to prevent diarrhea, symptoms of hypothyroidism appeared. Cholesterol level in the blood became elevated and in order to keep it within normal range, four additional grains of thyroid daily were needed. Apparently, a diet high in protein requires additional thyroid for its metabolism. There were no symptoms of hyperthyroidism in spite of the extra thyroid until the diet was cut back to a normal amount of protein. Then typical hyperthyroidism appeared and the extra thyroid had to be discontinued.

It seems clear that a diet quite high in protein utilizes available thyroid hormone. Two studies in the medical literature indicate that excess protein lowers the basal metabolism. This may explain why so few people have been successful in losing weight on the standard types of diets. With extra thyroid needed for utilization of protein, the metabolism could fall to the point that 800 calories a day would maintain existing weight rather than lead to weight loss.

This would also explain why some physicians specializing in weight reduction and using high-protein diets in their programs also use huge doses of thyroid without any apparent harm to their patients.

A Natural Approach to Obesity

It would appear that a rational and natural approach to overcoming obesity should employ a slightly modified diet containing approximately one gram of protein for each kilo (2.2 pounds) of body weight and a minimum of fifty grams of carbohydrate to avoid ketosis. Enough fat should then be added to keep the appetite satisfied and still not quite enough to satisfy the body needs, thus allowing a weight loss of one or two pounds a week. It may take a short time to adjust to the absence of excess carbohydrates previously consumed, but one can live on such a diet comfortably for long periods if some extra vitamin B is added.

Those who do not care enough about their health to follow such a diet program will probably suffer less damage by remaining overweight than by following crash diets.

16

The Role of the Thyroid in Aging

MAN WILL PROBABLY NEVER CEASE his search for (1) the stone of wisdom, (2) any easy source of unlimited wealth, and (3) the fountain of youth. All three are unattainable, the last certainly no less that the others. Yet much can be done to make the latter years of life more rewarding, less full of infirmities, both physical and mental.

Not long ago, Dr. Alexander Leaf of Harvard reported on his visits to and studies of three widely separated areas where many of the inhabitants not only live to advanced ages but remain vigorous and remarkably healthy even beyond the age of one hundred. One of these areas is in the Caucasus Mountains of Southern Russia, the second in the Land of Hunza in the Karakoram Range in Kashmir, and the third in the Andes Mountains in Ecuador.

276

Apparently, these three societies are spared much of the toll of infectious disease in the early years and, no less, much of the toll of degenerative diseases in later years. Many factors may be involved in the longevity and continued vigor in these societies. But an endowment of excellent thyroid function could well be one of the factors. For as we have seen, thyroid plays a major role in both resistance to infectious diseases and to the depradations of degenerative disorders and has much to do with the maintenance of mental health.

Just a few years before Dr. Leaf's report appeared, two Canadian physicians, Drs. J. P. Duruisseau and E. Laurendeau of the Hospital of Notre-Dame de la Merci in Montreal, published another on a study of thyroid function in elderly, chronically ill patients. The functioning of the thyroid, they found, had decreased in most of the patients. Moreover, treatment with thyroid extract resulted in noticeable clinical improvement in some of them. A decrease in thyroid function with age, they concluded, may be a cause of thyroid insufficiency and it may aggravate other conditions.

Thyroid function does commonly decrease with age. But low thyroid function is also common early in life and in mid-life. And whenever it occurs, it may contribute significantly to degenerative problems, and its correction may be of great benefit.

Where Degeneration Begins

In order to have systems with complex functions, there must be specialized cells. There must also be supporting structures for these complex systems—among them, for example, the blood vessel system and the nervous system. These supporting structures are usually of connective-tissue—and it is here where degeneration begins.

Between the cells in connective tissue is a "ground substance" which is concerned with the nutrition of the specialized cells. In thyroid-deficient patients, it is in the ground substance that mucopolysaccharides accumulate in abnormal quantities. Their affinity for fluid leads to swelling and pressure that may be destructive.

If the deposits accumulate in the ground substance in the connective tissue in the wall of a blood vessel, degenerative changes occur and atherosclerosis develops, restricting blood flow to the heart, the brain, the kidney, or other vital organs served by the blood vessel.

If the deposits are laid down in the ground substance in the connective tissue surrounding and supporting a nerve, the fluid accumulation and pressure may lead to tingling, numbness, or pain over the course of the nerve. If it is a motor nerve, the muscles supplied by that nerve may become weak or paralyzed.

Fortunately, if the thyroid deficiency is recognized early enough, thyroid therapy will cause the excess mucopolysaccharides to disappear, restoring normal function,

Any tissue in the body may be adversely affected by deposition of excess mucopolysaccharides resulting from hypothyroidism. For centuries, people living in the iodine-deficient areas of the Alps have appeared much older than their years. Mental deterioration among them was much more common than elsewhere.

Never Too Late

Low thyroid function, as we have noted, is common in young adulthood and even in childhood. It may become more pronounced with age. And, because thyroid function commonly decreases with age, hypothyroidism may only begin to develop in many cases in later years.

Whatever the age at which it occurs, it can produce the same symptoms, one, or several, or many: sensitivity to cold, susceptibility to infection, dry skin, falling hair, mental confusion, for example. And thyroid therapy can be beneficial at any age and may produce as dramatic effects at older ages as at younger.

Time after time, I have seen elderly patients respond. When one sixty-seven-year-old man sought help, his problems included rapidly developing baldness during the preceding year, a growing depletion of energy over the preceding two years, along with increasing forgetfulness, and increasingly severe mental depression. His physical examination disclosed elevated blood pressure, but nothing else. His basal temperature, however, was low. However easy it would have been to ascribe his various problems to senility and to dismiss him with an admonition to make the best of things, he was started on thyroid therapy with the suggestion that after a time this should make him feel better, but there was little hope of recovering his hair.

Two months later, when I saw him again, his depression had lifted, his blood pressure was down to normal, he was energetic, interested in life, and, to my own as well as his astonishment, hair was growing all over his head.

Frequently, both partners in a marriage are affected by problems that may seem on the surface to be due to aging and even senility. A sixty-eight-year-old woman complained of great fatigue and difficulty in swallowing. At that time, she was on digitalis for a failing heart and a potent antihypertensive medication. Her basal temperature indicated that the hypothyroidism had been present for much of her life.

She was started on one-half grain of thyroid which was later raised to a grain daily. Two months later, her difficulty in swallowing was gone, she felt well and full of energy, and no longer needed digitalis or the antihypertensive medicine.

Her husband came to me at the age of seventy, one year after he had had a heart attack. His history revealed that he had suffered for many years from migraine headaches, susceptibility to infections, constipation, and arthritis —all suggestive of hypothyroidism. His basal temperature was low.

He was started cautiously on thyroid, and the anticoagulant drug he had been taking was discontinued. Over the next few monthes, his energy level began to rise and he was soon able to discontinue his naps. As he continued thyroid, there was marked improvement in his headaches and other problems and he felt his health was improving greatly.

A year after he started thyroid therapy, he resumed fishing and not long afterward decided he was able to mow his own lawn again. Not long ago, I saw him and his wife, now aged seventy-eight and seventy-six, respectively, and both were full of vigor. They were accompanied by an adopted daughter and her husband and were heading for a camping trip. Eight years that might otherwise have been spent in failing health and restricted living had been turned into fruitful, happy living because the thermometer had indicated thyroid deficiency.

Not for one moment can it be assumed that thyroid deficiency is responsible for all the problems of senescence. It is more likely to be a factor in cases of premature senescence. Nor will even all of these respond dramatically to thyroid therapy. But the possibility that thyroid deficiency may be at work deserves careful consideration, and it costs nothing to take a basal temperature. If, indeed, thyroid function is shown to be low, thyroid therapy is simple and relatively inexpensive, and there is good chance it can make the remaining years far more pleasant.

17

A Word about Thyroid Treatment

THERE IS NOTHING DIFFICULT about correcting thyroid deficiency. It can be done effectively, inexpensively, and safely. The principles are simple, but it is essential that they be understood and followed.

In a person with normal thyroid function, when there is a need for more thyroid secretion, a signal is received by the pituitary gland which then releases a substance to stimulate thyroid function. As soon as the needed amount of thyroid secretion has then been released into the bloodstream, the pituitary gland gets the message, stops releasing its thyroid-stimulating substance, and less thyroid is produced. Through this sensitive "feedback" mechanism, the amount of thyroid hormone in the bloodstream is maintained in an effective, narrow range.

When thyroid function is deficient, the gland cannot respond adequately to the stimulus from the pituitary.

Then, it is necessary to supply a small amount of thyroid hormone from the outside, just as insulin from the outside is supplied for the diabetic.

But remember the feedback mechanism. If an excess of thyroid is supplied from the outside, the pituitary gland will get the signal that there is such an excess and will stop its stimulus to the thyroid gland, and thyroid function may be depressed still further. With sufficient excess supplied from the outside, the thyroid may stop putting out any hormone. In that case, all thyroid is coming from the outside; the body's precise control of thyroid level in the bloodstream is thwarted; and it is possible that the patient may even have too much hormone in the blood and may develop some or many of the symptoms of hyperthyroidism such as nervousness, sleeping difficulty, excessive sweating, elevated temperature, and loss of weight.

None of this is necessary. If a small dose is used to begin with and the dose is raised only if necessary—and, then, gradually—the thyroid gland will continue to function as it has before, its deficiency will be overcome, the feedback mechanism will be maintained intact, and the amount of thyroid in the bloodstream will be kept in the effective, narrow range found in people with normal thyroid function.

At the Start

The size of a proper starting dose of thyroid will vary with the age and size of the patient. Usually a child under three years of age will not need more than one-quarter grain daily. By the age of six, one-half grain may be used in the beginning. A teen-ager or adult may safely be started on one grain daily. For a particularly large man or woman, two grains may be used—but no more than that at the beginning. The starting dosage should be maintained for about two months. After that, if necessary, the dosage may be increased.

An important caution: Anyone who has had a heart attack should not be started on thyroid therapy for at least two months afterward. Then the starting dose should not be greater than one-half grain a day. During thyroid therapy, the heart is called upon to do a little more work. It is normal, healthy work and can benefit the heart—but the heart is not ready for it for a time after a heart attack and when the time is ripe, at about two months after the attack, the work must be increased slowly.

When the Benefits Begin

Thyroid therapy does not produce overnight change. No change may be noted for about a month. Usually, at some point between one month and two months after the beginning of therapy, some of the symptoms begin to subside and the individual begins to feel better. At that point, an evaluation is in order to determine whether the starting dosage is sufficient for continued use or if an increase in dosage is advisable.

If all symptoms have disappeared, the individual feels in good physical and mental health, and is adjusting well to work and other normal activities, the same dosage may be continued. If symptoms have improved to some extent but have not disappeared entirely, an increase in dosage may be needed. If the blood cholesterol was high to begin with and has fallen to some extent but not to normal, the dosage may be increased if the basal temperature is still low.

When an increase in dosage is indicated, the amount of the increase again depends upon age and size of the individual. In children, not more than one-quarter grain should be added to the initial dosage. In the teen-ager, the increment should be one-half grain. In the adult as much as one grain should be added. The new dosage should be continued for two months, at which time another evaluation should be done. If necessary, at this point, the dosage may be increased again, and again the increment is the same as for the previous increase.

The proper dosage for any individual is the minimum needed to relieve symptoms. Most commonly, in adults, this is two grains; three grains sometimes are needed, rarely four grains may be required. The basal temperature may still be a little low, but one is treating symptoms, not temperature per se.

The Guide

The basal temperature can serve as an excellent guide not only to the need for thyroid therapy but also to achieving the proper thyroid dosage. The normal range of basal termperature is between 97.8 and 98.2 degrees Fahrenheit. When symptoms of thyroid deficiency are present, the basal temperature may be one, two, or even three degrees below normal. With thyroid therapy, the temperature will start to rise.

During treatment, it should not exceed the upper limit of normal—98.2—unless a cold, sore throat, or other infection is present. The thyroid gland will not decrease its normal function unless the basal temperature is maintained for some time above the upper limit of normal.

One mistake which has been made in the past has been to start thyroid therapy with excessive amounts. Another has been to give up too soon—to expect immediate results, immediate disappearance of symptoms. And still a third has been to stop thyroid therapy because the patient has become nervous and the nervousness has been thought to be the result of too much thyroid.

All three of these mistakes can be avoided with use of the basal temperature as a guide, starting with the dosages already recommended, noting the effects on both symptoms and basal temperature, and adjusting the dosage to bring the temperature closer to the normal range.

Anyone can become nervous for many reasons other than too much thyroid. Financial difficulties, job frustrations, marital problems, and other anxiety-provoking or tension-building situations may lead to symptoms mimicking those of excessive thyroid activity. If the basal temperature is still low or within the normal range, it is a clear indication that the nervousness and other symptoms are not coming from too much thyroid and thyroid therapy should continue while an effort is made to overcome or adjust to what is really the disturbing factor.

Bibliography

CHAPTER 1

Barnes, Broda O., and Barnes, Charlotte W. *Heart Attack Rareness in Thyroid-Treated Patients*. Charles C. Thomas, Springfield, Illinois, 1972, page 30.

Crispell, K.R. *Current Concepts in Hypothyroidism*. The Macmillan Company, New York, 1963.

Means, J.H.; DeGroot, L.J.; and Stanbury, J.B. *The Thyroid and Its Diseases*, 3rd ed. McGraw-Hill, New York, 1963.

Pitt-Rivers, R., and Trotter, W.R. *The Thyroid Gland*, Vols. I and II. Butterworths, London, 1964.

Werner, S.C., and Ingbar, S.H. *The Thyroid*. Harper & Row, New York, 1971.

Williams, R.H. *Textbook of Endocrinology*. W.B. Saunders, Philadelphia, 1968.

CHAPTER 2

Barnes, Broda O., and Barnes, Charlotte W. *Heart Attack Rareness in Thyroid-Treated Patients.* Charles C. Thomas, Springfield, Illinois, 1972, page 30.

Means, J.H.; DeGroot, L.J.; and Stanbury, J.B. *The Thyroid and Its Diseases.* McGraw-Hill, New York, 1963, pages 321–322.

Starr, P. *Hypothyroidism.* Charles C. Thomas, Springfield, Illinois, 1954, page 46.

CHAPTER 3

Barnes, Broda O., and Barnes, Charlotte W. *Heart Attack Rareness in Thyroid-Treated Patients.* Charles C. Thomas, Springfield, Illinois, 1972, page 58.

Basinger, H.R. "The Control of Experimental Cretinism," in *Archives Internal Medicine,* 17:1916, page 260.

Jackson, A.S. "Hypothyroidism," in *JAMA,* 165:121, 1957.

Kimball, O.P. "Clinical Hypothyroidism," in *Kentucky Medical Journal,* 31:488, 1933.

Wharton, G.K. "Unrecognized Hypothyroidism," in *Canadian Medical Association Journal,* 40:371, 1939.

CHAPTER 4

Means, J.H. "Circulatory Disturbances in Diseases of the Glands of Internal Secretion," in *Endocrinology,* 9:192, 1925.

Stewart, H.J.; Dietrick, J.E.; and Crane, N.F. "Studies of the Circulation in Patients Suffering from Spontaneous Myxedema," in *Journal of Clinical Investigation,* 17:237, 1938.

CHAPTER 5

Barnes, Broda O. "Headache—Etiology and Treatment," in *Federation Proceedings,* 6:73, 1947.

CHAPTER 6

Ashner, R. "Myxedematous Madness," in *British Medical Journal,* 2:555, 1949.

Bruns, Report of a committee of the Clinical Society of London to investigate the subject of myxoedema. *Transactions Clinical Society London,* supplement to Vol. 21, 1888, page 105.

Cremer, G.M., et al. *Neurology,* 19:37.

Murray, G.R.; Allbut, C.; Rolleston, A.D. "Myxoedema," in *A System of Medicine.* Macmillan and Company, London, 1908.

Prange, A.J., Jr.; Wilson, I.C.; Rabon, A.M.; and Lipton, M.A. "Enhancement of Imipramine Activity by Thyroid Hormone," in *American Journal Psychiatry,* 126:457, 1969.

Sanders, V. "Neurologic Manifestations of Myxedema," in *New England Journal of Medicine,* 226:599, 1962.

Schon, M. "Untreated Thyroid Deficiency and Psychologic Disorders," Report to American Psychological Association, 72nd annual convention, Los Angeles.

Smith, C.A.; Oberhelman, H.A.; Storer, E.H.; Woodward, E.R.; and Dragstedt, L.R. "Production of Experimental Cretinism in Dogs by the Administration of Radioactive Iodine," in *Archives Surgery,* 63:807, 1951.

Whybrow, M.B.; Prange, A.J., Jr.; and Treadway, C.R. "Mental Changes Accompanying Thyroid Gland Dysfunction," in *Archives General Psychiatry,* 20:48, 1969.

Report of a Committee of the Clinical Society of London to investigate the subject of myxoedema. *Transactions Clinical Society London,* supplement to Vol. 21, 1888.

CHAPTER 7

Barnes, Broda O. "Etiology and Treatment of Lowered Resistance to Upper Respiratory Infection," in *Federation Proceedings,* 12:10, 1953.

White, Paul Dudley. *Heart Disease.* The Macmillan Company, New York, 1937.

CHAPTER 8

Andersen, H.; Asboe-Hansen, G.; and Quaade, F. "Histopathologic Examination of the Skin in the Diagnosis of Myxedema in Children," in *Journal Clinical Endocrinology,* 15:459, 1955.

Asboe-Hansen, G. "The Variability in the Hyaluronic Acid Content of the Dermal Connective Tissue under the Influence of the Thyroid Hormone," in *Acta derm-venerol,* 30:221, 1950.

Barnes, Broda O. "Furunculosis—Etiology and Treatment," in *Journal Clinical Endocrinology,* 3:243, 1943.

————"Thyroid Therapy in Dermatology," in *Cutis,* December 1971.

Bramwell, B. "A Clinical Lecture on a Case of Psoriasis Treated by Thyroid Extract," in *British Medical Journal,* 1:617, 1894.

Gull, W. "A Cretinoid State Supervening in the Adult Life of Women," in *London Clinical Society Transactions,* 7:180–185, 1875.

Horsley, V. "The Thyroid Gland," in *British Medical Journal,* 1:211, 1885.

Ord, W.M. "On Myxoedema, a Term Proposed to be Applied to an Essential Condition in the Cretinoid Infection Occasionally Observed in Middle-aged Women," in *Trans Med-Churg Society London,* 60–61:57–78, 1877–78.

Stewart, H.J., and Evans, W.F. "Peripheral Blood Flow in Myxedema," in *Archives Internal Medicine*, 69:808, 1942.

Sutton, R.L. *Diseases of the Skin.* C.V. Mosby, St. Louis, 1956.

CHAPTER 9

Barnes, Broda O. "The Treatment of Menstrual Disorders in General Practice," in *Arizona Medicine*, 6:33, 1949.

Foster, R.C., and Thornton, M.J. "Thyroid in Treatment of Menstrual Irregularities," in *Endocrinology*, 24:383, 1939.

Litzenberg, J.C. "The Endocrines in Relation to Sterility and Abortion," in *JAMA*, 109:1871, 1937.

Means, J.H. *The Thyroid and Its Diseases*, 2nd ed. Lippincott, Philadelphia, 1948, page 571.

Ross, G.T.; Scholz, D.A.; Lambert, F.H.; and Geraci, J.E. "Severe Uterine Bleeding and Degenerative-Skeletal Muscle Changes in Unrecognized Myxedema," in *Journal Clinical Endocrinology and Metabolism*, 18:492, 1958.

Scott, J.C. Jr., and Mussey, E. "Menstrual Patterns in Myxedema," in *American Journal Obstetrics and Gynecology*, 90:161, 1965.

Silenkow, H.R., and Refetoff, S. "Common Tests of Thyroid Function in Serum," in *JAMA*, 202:135, 1967.

Report of a committee of the Clinical Society of London to investigate the subject of myxoedema. *Transactions Clinical Society London*, supplement to Vol. 21, 1888.

CHAPTER 10

Fishberg, A.M. "Arteriosclerosis in Thyroid Deficiency," in *JAMA* 82:463, 1924.

Goldblatt, H. "Studies on Experimental Hypertension," in *Annals Internal Medicine*, 11:69, 1937.

Menof, P. "New Method for Control of Hypertension," in *South African Medical Journal,* 24:172, 1950.

Ord, W.M. "On Myxoedema, a Term Proposed to be Applied to an Essential Condition in the Cretinoid Infection Occasionally Observed in Middle-aged Women." *Trans Med-Churg Society London,* 60–61:57–78, 1877–78.

CHAPTER 11

Barnes, Broda O.; and Barnes, Charlotte W. *Heart Attack Rareness in Thyroid-Treated Patients.* Charles C. Thomas, Springfield, Illinois, 1972, page 30.

Barnes, Broda O.; Ratzenhofer, M.; Gisi, R. "The Role of Natural Consequences in the Changing Death Patterns," in *Journal American Geriatric Society,* 22:176, 1974.

Christian, H.A. "The Heart and Its Management in Myxedema," in *Rhode Island Medical Journal,* 8:109, 1925.

Dawber, T.R.; Moore, F.E.; and Mann, G.V. "Coronary Heart Disease in the Framingham Study," in *American Journal Public Health,* 47:4–24, 1957.

DeLangen, C.D. "Cholesterol Metabolism and Racial Pathology," (In Dutch, "Gencesk Tijdschr. v. Nederl") Indie, 56,1, 1916.

Falta, W. *Endocrine Diseases,* 3rd ed., Translated by Milton K. Myers. P. Blakiston's Son and Company, Philadelphia, 1923.

Higginson, J., and Pepler, W.J. "Fat Intake, Serum Cholesterol Concentration and Atherosclerosis in the South African Bantu," in *Part II, Atherosclerosis and Coronary Artery Disease. Journal Clinical Investigation,* 33:1366, 1954.

Hurxthal, L.M. "Blood Cholesterol and Thyroid Disease," in *Archives Internal Medicine,* 53:762, 1934.

Israel, M. "An Effective Therapeutic Approach to the Control of Atherosclerosis Illustrating Harmlessness of Prolonged Use of Thyroid Hormone in Coronary Disease," in *American Journal Digestive Diseases,* 22:161–168, 1955.

Kimura, N. "Analysis of 10,000 Postmortem Examinations in Japan." *World Trends in Cardiology,* Vol. 1. *Cardiovascular Epidemiology,* Hoeber-Harper, New York, 1956, page 159.

Kountz, W.B. *Thyroid Function and Its Possible Role in Vascular Degeneration.* Charles C. Thomas, Springfield, Illinois, 1951.

Laurie, W.; Woods, J.D.; and Roach, G. "Coronary Heart Disease in the South African Bantu," in *American Journal Cardiology,* 5:48–59, 1960.

Leary, T. "Experimental Atherosclerosis in the Rabbit Compared with Human (Coronary) Atherosclerosis," in *Archives Pathology,* 17:453–492, 1934.

Lerman, J., and White, Paul Dudley. "Metabolic Changes in Young People with Coronary Heart Disease," in *Journal Clinical Investigation,* 25:914, 1946 (Proceedings).

Lidsky, A., and Kottman, K. "Influence of the Thyroids on Blood Clotting," in *Zeitschrift klin Medicin,* 71:344, 1911.

Malysheva, L.V. "Tissue Respiration Rate in Certain Organs in Experimental Hypercholesterolemia and Atherosclerosis," in *Federation Proceedings Translation Supplement,* 23:T562, 1964.

Ord, W.M. "On Myxoedema, a Term Proposed to Be Applied to an Essential Condition in the Cretinoid Infection Occasionally Observed in Middle-aged Women," in *Transactions Med-Churg Society London,* 60–61; 57–78, 1877–78.

Smyth, C.J. "Angina Pectoris and Myocardial Infarction as Complications of Myxedema," in *American Heart Journal,* 15:652–660, 1938.

Strisower, B.; Gofman, J.W.; Gaglioni, E.; Ribinger, J.; O'Brien, G.W.; and Simon, A. "Effects of Long-Term Administration of Desiccated Thyroid on Serum Lipoprotein and Cholesterol Level," in *Journal Clinical Endocrinology,* 15:73–80, 1955.

Sturgis, C.C., and Whiting, W.B. "The Treatment and Prognosis in Myxedema," in *JAMA,* 85:2013, 1925.

Turner, K.B.; Present, C.H.; and Bidwell, E.H. "The Role of Thyroid in the Regulation of the Blood Cholesterol in Rabbits," in *Journal Experimental Medicine,* 67:111, 1938.

Virchow, Rudolf. "Genauere geschichte der fittmetamorphose," The Cellularpathologic Berlin 1858 Verlog von August Hirschwald.

von Eiselsberg, A.F. "On Vegetative Disturbances in Growth of Animals after Early Thyroidectomy," in *Archives Klinik Chirugie,* 49:207, 1895.

Wren, J.C. "Thyroid Function and Coronary Atherosclerosis," *Journal American Geriatric Society,* 16:696–704, 1968.

Zondek, H. "The Myxedema Heart," in *Munchen Medical Worchenschrift,* 65:1180, 1918.

Report of a committee of the Clinical Society of London to investigate the subject of myxoedema. *Transactions Clinical Society London,* supplement to Vol. 21, 1888.

CHAPTER 12

Andersen, H.; Asboe-Hansen, G.; and Quaade, F. "Histopathologic Examination of the Skin in the Diagnosis of Myxedema in Children," in *Journal Clinical Investigation,* 15:459, 1955.

Asboe-Hansen, G. "The Variability in the Hyaluronic Acid Content of the Dermal Connective Tissue under the Influence of Thyroid Hormone," in *Acta derm-venerology*, 30:221, 1950.

Golding, P.N. "Hypothyroidism Presenting with Muscolo-Skeletal Symptoms," in *Annals Rheumatic Diseases*, 29:10, 1970.

Hill, S.R.; Reiss, R.S.; Forsham, P.H.; and Thorn, G.W. "The Effect of Adrenocorticotropin and Cortisone on Thyroid Function; Thyroid-Adrenocortical Interrelationships," in *Journal Clinical Endocrinology*, 10:1375, 1950.

Horsley, V. "The Thyroid Gland," in *British Medical Journal*, 1:111, 1885.

Ord, W.M. "On Myxoedema, a Term Proposed to Be Applied to an Essential Condition in the Cretinoid Infection Occasionally Observed in Middle-aged Women," in *Trans Med-Churg Society London*, 60–61:57–78, 1877–78.

Swain, L.T. "Chronic Arthritis," in *JAMA*, 93:259, 1929.

CHAPTER 13

Banting, F.G., and Best, Charles. "The Internal Secretion of the Pancreas," in *Journal Laboratory Clinical Medicine*, 7:251, 1922.

Barnes, Broda O., and Regan, J.F. "The Relation of the Anterior Pituitary to Carbohydrate Metabolism," in *Endocrinology*, 17:522, 1933.

Eaton, C.D. "Coexistance of Hypothyroidism with Diabetes Mellitus," in *Journal Michigan Medical Society*, 53:1101, 1954.

Ellenberg, M. "Diabetic Complications Without Manifest Diabetes: Complications as Presenting Clinical Symptoms," in *JAMA*, 183:926, 1963.

Gardiner-Hill, H.; Brett, A.C.; and Smith, J.F. "Carbohydrate Tolerance in Myxedema," in *Quarterly Journal Medicine*, 18:327, 1925.

Jackson, W.P.V. "The Expression 'Prediabetes'," in *Diabetes,* 11:334, 1962.

Joslin, E.P. "Arteriosclerosis in Diabetes," in *Annals Internal Medicine,* 4:54, 1930.

Lukens, F.D.W., and Franklin, S.N. "Long-Term Diabetes Without Vascular Disease," in *Medical Clinics North America,* 50:1385, 1966.

Moses, C.; Danowski, T.S.; and Switkes, H.E. "Alterations in Cholesterol and Lipoprotein Partition in Euthroid Adults by Replacement Doses of Desiccated Thyroid," in *Circulation,* 18:761, 1958.

Prout, T.E., and Goldner, M.G. "The University Group Diabetes Program," in *Diabetes,* 19:(supplement 1) 375, 1970.

Schaefer, O. "Glucose Tolerance Testing in Canadian Eskimos: A Preliminary Report and a Hypothesis," in *Canadian Medical Association Journal,* 99:252, 1968.

CHAPTER 14

Barnes, B.O., and Ratzenhofer, M. "One Factor in Increase of Bronchial Carcinoma," in *JAMA,* 174:2229, 1960.

Campbell, R.E., and Hughes, F.A. "The Development of Bronchiogenic Carcinoma in Patients with Pulmonary Tuberculosis," in *Journal Thoracic and Cardiovascular Surgery,* 40:98, 1960.

Duguid, J.B. "The Incidence of Intra-Thoracic Tumours in Manchester," in *Lancet* 2:111, 1927.

Spencer, J.G.C. "The Influence of the Thyroid in Malignant Disease," in *British Journal of Cancer,* 8:393, 1954.

Williams, W.R. "Remarks on the Mortality from Cancer," in *Lancet* 2:481, 1898.

Wolf, K. "The Primary Lung Cancer," in *Fortschritte d Medicin,* 13:725, 1895.

CHAPTER 15

Anderson, A.B. "Loss of Weight in Obese Patients on Sub-Maintenance Diets and the Effect of Variation in the Ratio of Carbohydrate to Fat in the Diet," in *Quarterly Journal Medicine,* 13:27, 1944.

Barnes, Broda O. "A Practical Diet for Weight Reduction," in *Federation Proceedings,* 24:314, 1965.

Duncan, T.G. "The Burden of Obesity," in *Internist Observer,* October-November 1970.

Evans, F.A., and Strang, J.M. "A Departure from the Usual Methods in Treating Obesity," in *American Journal of Medical Science,* 177:339, 1929.

Keckwick, A., and Pawan, G.L.S. "Caloric Intake in Relation to Body-Weight Changes in the Obese," in *Lancet* 2:155, 1956.

Lieb, C.W. "The Effects on Human Beings of a Twelve-Month's Exclusive Meat Diet," in *JAMA,* 93:20, 1929; *Journal Biological Chemistry,* 87:651, 1930; *Journal Biological Chemistry,* 83:753, 1929.

Pennington, A.W. "The Use of Fat in a Weight-Reducing Diet," in *Delaware State Medical Journal,* 23:79, 1951.

Index

acne, 9, 105-107
adrenal glands, 18, 223
  cholesterol in, 169
  cortisone and, 205
  tumor of, 144
adrenaline, 18
aging, thyroid function in, 276-281
  longevity and, 276-277
  mucopolysaccharides and, 278
alcohol, heart and, 158
allergy, 22-23
alveoli, 248, 250
Andersen, Karsten, 272
Anderson, A. B., 266
Anderson, H., 109
anemia, 20, 26, 57-60
anginal pain, 165, 187, 250
Anitschkow, N., 170, 172
antibiotics, 97, 103, 104, 250

antibiotics (cont.)
  and death from infection, 160, 251
  as rheumatic fever preventative,
    94-95
antibodies, 90
antidepressant drugs, 80
antihypertensive medication, 145,
    152-153
aorta, narrowing of, 144
Armour Tech students,
  hypothyroidism in, 39, 76-78
armpit (axillary) temperature, 45-46
artery lining, cholesterol and, 171
arthritis, 197-213
  cortisone and, 205-207
  fever in, 205
  gouty, 212-213
  infection and, 203
  pain of, 197

Index